Surgery

NOTICE

Surgery

PreTest® Self-Assessment and Review

Fifth Edition

Edited by

Thomas C. King, M.D.
Ferrer Professor of Surgery
College of Physicians and Surgeons
Columbia University
New York, New York

Peter L. Geller, M.D.
Assistant Professor of Surgery
College of Physicians and Surgeons
Columbia University
New York, New York

Paul M. Starker, M.D.
Assistant Professor of Surgery
College of Physicians and Surgeons
Columbia University
New York, New York

McGraw-Hill Information Services Company
Health Professions Division
PreTest Series

New York St. Louis San Francisco Colorado Springs Auckland Bogotá Hamburg Lisbon London Madrid Mexico Milan Montreal New Delhi Panama Paris San Juan São Paulo Singapore Sydney Tokyo Toronto

Library of Congress Cataloging-in-Publication Data

Surgery : PreTest self-assessment and review.

Bibliography: p.
1. Surgery—Examinations, questions, etc.
I. King, Thomas C., 1928– . II. Geller, Peter L. III.
III. Starker, Paul M. [DNLM: 1. Surgery—examination questions. WL 18 S959]
RD37.2.S97 1989 617'.0076 88–27149
ISBN 0-07-051974-9

This book was set in Times Roman by Waldman Graphics, Inc.; the editors were J. Dereck Jeffers and Bruce MacGregor; the production supervisor was Clara B. Stanley.
R. R. Donnelley & Sons was printer and binder.

1 2 3 4 5 6 7 8 9 0 DOCDOC 8 9 4 3 2 1 0 9

ISBN 0-07-051974-9

Contents

Contributors

John A. Chabot, M.D.
Senior Resident in General Surgery
Columbia-Presbyterian Medical Center
New York, New York

Timothy A. M. Chuter, M.D.
Senior Resident in General Surgery
Columbia-Presbyterian Medical Center
New York, New York

David W. Johnstone, M.D.
Senior Resident in General Surgery
Columbia-Presbyterian Medical Center
New York, New York

Mehmet C. Oz, M.D.
Senior Resident in General Surgery
Columbia-Presbyterian Medical Center
New York, New York

Preface

Although the questions—and explanations—presented in this book are designed chiefly as a review in preparation for certifying examinations, the approach they embody has much to recommend it as a study format in a more general sense. The lives of physicians are made up of a series of real problems, the solutions of which require a series of logical steps: analyzing patient-related data; recalling relevant information, both general and specific; making choices among alternatives; reviewing the consequences of action taken; and making corrections in plans. The problem-solving model, as a stimulus to studying and learning, simulates to a small degree this learning model. It also takes advantage of many of the characteristics recognized by educational psychologists as conducive to efficient learning experiences. Information is gathered in response to a perceived need rather than in anticipation of that need. The learner is actively involved. There is immediate feedback, error correction, and reinforcement. The process can be carried out at the learner's own pace and in a natural setting. The material in this book is an approach to continuing education of student-physicians using methods designed to exploit these characteristics.

No longer can students assume that this kind of continuing education ends with the completion of formal training and the successful completion of licensing or certifying examinations. As of October 1979, all 22 member boards of the American Board of Medical Specialties had committed themselves to the principle of periodic recertification of their members. Despite the Board's recognition that the cognitive skills measured in the objective examination do not assure clinical competence, recertification efforts—insofar as they involve examinations—are based on the assumption that knowledge of current information upon which good clinical decisions should be made is worth cultivating; that, while such information does not guarantee competent practice, lack of it probably impedes competent practice; that this knowledge, unlike technical skills, is reasonably easy to assess, and that it can be acquired by well-motivated physicians. These assumptions all seem reasonable.

The questions presented in this book deal with issues of relative importance to medical students; other problem-oriented materials are becoming available that are aimed at more sophisticated audiences—groups that, within a very few years, will include the present generation of students. Regular review of such material is a habit worth developing. We hope that this edition of *Surgery, PreTest Self-Assessment and Review* will justify your efforts in working through the problems by providing guidance for further study and helping to develop enduring learning habits.

Thomas C. King, M.D.

Introduction

Surgery, PreTest Self-Assessment and Review, 5th Ed., has been designed to provide medical students, as well as physicians, with a comprehensive and convenient instrument for self-assessment and review within the field of surgery. The 500 questions provided have the same format and are of the same degree of difficulty as the questions contained in Part II of the National Board of Medical Examiners examinations, the Federation Licensing Examination (FLEX), and the Foreign Medical Graduate Examination in the Medical Sciences (FMGEMS).

Each question in the book is accompanied by an answer, a paragraph explanation, and a specific page reference to either a current journal article, a textbook, or both. A bibliography, which lists all the sources used in the book, follows the last chapter.

Perhaps the most effective way to use this book is to allow yourself one minute to answer each question in a given chapter; as you proceed, indicate your answer beside each question. By following this suggestion, you will be approximating the time limits imposed by the board examinations previously mentioned.

When you have finished answering the questions in a chapter, you should then spend as much time as you need verifying your answers and carefully reading the explanations. Although you should pay special attention to the explanations for the questions you answered incorrectly, you should read every explanation. The authors of this book have designed the explanations to reinforce and supplement the information tested by the questions. If, after reading the explanations for a given chapter, you feel you need still more information about the material covered, you should consult and study the references indicated.

Surgery

Pre- and Postoperative Care

DIRECTIONS: Each question below contains five suggested responses. Select the **one best** response to each question.

1. The earliest clinical indication of hypermagnesemia is

(A) loss of deep tendon reflexes
(B) flaccid paralysis
(C) respiratory arrest
(D) hypotension
(E) stupor

2. Hyponatremia may result from all the following clinical problems EXCEPT

(A) diuretic abuse
(B) diabetes insipidus
(C) the nephrotic syndrome
(D) cirrhosis
(E) adrenal insufficiency

3. In the management of severe hypercalcemia, all the following agents are useful EXCEPT

(A) thiazide diuretics
(B) furosemide
(C) prednisone
(D) mithramycin
(E) infused phosphate

4. A 45-year-old woman with Crohn's disease and a small intestinal fistula develops tetany during the second week of parenteral nutrition. The laboratory findings include Ca 8.2 mEq/L, Na 135 mEq/L, K 3.2 mEq/L, Cl 103 mEq/L, P_{O_4} 2.4 mEq/L, albumin 2.4, pH 7.48, P_{CO_2} 38 torr, P_{O_2} 84 torr, and bicarbonate 25 mEq/L. The most likely cause of her tetany is

(A) hyperventilation
(B) hypocalcemia
(C) hypomagnesemia
(D) essential fatty acid deficiency
(E) focal seizure

5. Which of the following is characteristic of hypernatremia?

(A) Dry, sticky, oral mucous membranes
(B) Decreased body temperature
(C) Decreased deep tendon reflexes
(D) Stupor and coma
(E) None of the above

6. You are modifying a standard total parenteral nutrition (TPN) solution for a patient in renal failure. All the following should be eliminated or given in reduced quantities EXCEPT

(A) total volume
(B) potassium
(C) magnesium
(D) phosphate
(E) calcium

Questions 7–8

A previously healthy 55-year-old man undergoes elective cholecystectomy for asymptomatic cholelithiasis. His postoperative ileus is somewhat prolonged, and on the fifth postoperative day his nasogastric tube is still in place. Physical examination reveals diminished skin turgor, dry mucous membranes, and orthostatic hypotension. Pertinent laboratory values are as follow:

Arterial blood gases: pH 7.56; P_{O_2} 85 torr; P_{CO_2} 50 torr
Serum electrolytes (mEq/L): Na^+ 132, K^+ 3.1; Cl^- 80; HCO_3^- 42
Urine electrolytes (mEq/L): Na^+ 2; K^- 5; Cl^- 6

7. The values given above allow the descriptive diagnosis of

(A) uncompensated metabolic alkalosis
(B) respiratory acidosis with metabolic compensation
(C) combined metabolic alkalosis
(D) metabolic alkalosis with respiratory compensation
(E) "paradoxical" metabolic respiratory alkalosis

8. The most appropriate therapy for the patient described would be

(A) infusion of 0.9% NaCl with supplemental KCl until clinical signs of volume depletion are eliminated
(B) infusion of isotonic (0.15 *N*) HCl via a central venous catheter
(C) clamping the nasogastric tube to prevent further acid losses
(D) administration of acetazolamide to promote renal excretion of bicarbonate
(E) intubation and controlled hypoventilation on a volume-cycled ventilator to further increase the P_{CO_2}

9. A 27-year-old woman is hospitalized in stage IV coma after an automobile accident. She is found to have cerebrospinal fluid otorrhea. A few hours later she begins to void large volumes of hypotonic urine (400 ml/hr, specific gravity 1.003 to 1.005). The most appropriate management for this patient is

(A) replacement of urinary losses with 0.9% NaCl
(B) replacement of urinary losses with 5% glucose in water
(C) administration of subcutaneous aqueous vasopressin, 5 U
(D) administration of intramuscular vasopressin tannate in oil, 5 U
(E) observation

Questions 10–11

A 23-year-old woman is brought to the emergency room from a halfway house, where she had apparently swallowed a handful of pills. The patient complains of shortness of breath and tinnitus, but refuses to identify the pills she ingested. Pertinent laboratory values are as follow:

Arterial blood gases: pH 7.45; P_{O_2} 126 torr; P_{CO_2} 12 torr
Serum electrolytes (mEq/L): Na^+ 138; K^+ 4.8; Cl^- 102; HCO_3^- 8

10. The patient's acid-base disturbance is best characterized by which of the following descriptions?

(A) Acute respiratory alkalosis, compensated
(B) Chronic respiratory alkalosis, compensated
(C) Metabolic acidosis, compensated
(D) Mixed metabolic acidosis and respiratory alkalosis
(E) Mixed metabolic acidosis and respiratory acidosis

11. The most likely cause of the disturbance in this patient is an overdose of

(A) phenformin
(B) aspirin
(C) barbiturates
(D) methanol
(E) diazepam (Valium)

12. A 37-year-old woman with severe Crohn's disease receives 1 month of TPN prior to undergoing a small bowel resection. Two weeks postoperatively she develops a facial rash and begins complaining that her hair is falling out. Her skin sutures are removed and the wound separates. A deficiency of which of the following should be suspected?

(A) Essential fatty acids
(B) Chromium
(C) Magnesium
(D) Zinc
(E) None of the above

13. A 68-year-old man is admitted to the coronary care unit with an acute myocardial infarction. His postinfarction course is marked by congestive heart failure and intermittent hypotension. On the fourth hospital day, he develops severe midabdominal pain. On physical examination, blood pressure is 90/60 mmHg, pulse 110/min and regular; the abdomen is soft with mild generalized tenderness and distention. Bowel sounds are hypoactive; stool hematest is positive. The next step in this patient's management should be which of the following?

(A) Barium enema
(B) Upper gastrointestinal series
(C) Angiography
(D) Ultrasonography
(E) Celiotomy

14. All the following are risk factors for perioperative myocardial infarction EXCEPT

(A) coronary artery bypass 3 months prior to the current procedure
(B) a third heart sound
(C) old age (in the absence of any history of cardiac disease)
(D) myocardial infarction 1 year prior to the current procedure
(E) a non–Q-wave myocardial infarction 3 weeks prior to emergency surgery

15. A 20-year-old woman is found to have an activated partial thromboplastin time (APTT) of 78/32 on routine testing prior to cholecystectomy. Further investigation reveals a prothrombin time (PT) of 13/12 (patient/control), a template bleeding time of 13 min, and a platelet count of $350 \times 100/\text{mm}^3$. All the following are true of this woman's coagulopathy EXCEPT

(A) infusion of factor VIII concentrate is usually required to normalize concentration prior to surgery
(B) transfusion of cryoprecipitate will be followed by an improvement in coagulation
(C) few of these patients are seropositive for HIV
(D) epistaxis or menorrhagia is common
(E) lack of aggregation in response to ristocetin is a common feature of this disease

16. A 30-year-old woman in the last trimester of pregnancy suddenly develops massive left lower extremity swelling from the inguinal ligament to the ankle. The correct sequence of workup and treatment should be

(A) venogram, bed rest, heparin
(B) impedance plethysmography, bed rest, heparin
(C) impedance plethysmography, bed rest, vena caval filter
(D) impedance plethysmography, bed rest, heparin, warfarin (Coumadin)
(E) clinical evaluation, bed rest, warfarin

17. The chief surgical risk to which patients with polycythemia vera are exposed is that due to

(A) anemic disturbances
(B) hemorrhage
(C) infection
(D) renal dysfunction
(E) cardiopulmonary complications

18. Banked blood is deficient in which of the following coagulation factors?

(A) II only
(B) II and VII
(C) V and VIII
(D) IX and X
(E) XI and XII

19. A 25-year-old woman underwent subtotal thyroidectomy for Graves' disease. Postoperatively she noticed that her voice fatigued easily and that she became hoarse when she talked for long periods. The most probable cause of her dysphonia is

(A) injury to the vagus nerve
(B) injury to the recurrent laryngeal nerve
(C) injury to the superior laryngeal nerve
(D) persistent perilaryngeal postoperative infection
(E) an emotional reaction

DIRECTIONS: Each question below contains four suggested responses of which **one or more** is correct. Select

A	if	**1, 2, and 3**	are correct
B	if	**1 and 3**	are correct
C	if	**2 and 4**	are correct
D	if	**4**	is correct
E	if	**1, 2, 3, and 4**	are correct

20. Reduction of an elevated potassium level can be obtained by use of

(1) sodium polystyrene sulfonate (Kayexalate)
(2) sodium bicarbonate
(3) glucose and insulin
(4) calcium gluconate

21. A 23-year-old woman undergoes total thyroidectomy for carcinoma of the thyroid gland. On the second postoperative day she begins to complain of tingling sensation in her hands. She appears quite anxious and later complains of muscle cramps. Appropriate therapy over the next several days might include administration of

(1) 10 ml of 10% calcium chloride intravenously
(2) continuous infusion of calcium gluconate
(3) oral calcium gluconate
(4) oral vitamin D

22. Patients on long-term hyperalimentation may develop deficiencies in which of the following nutrients because of their insolubility in solution?

(1) Vitamin K
(2) Vitamin A
(3) Folic Acid
(4) Ascorbic Acid

23. A 43-year-old woman develops acute renal failure following an emergency resection of a leaking abdominal aortic aneurysm. Three days after surgery, the following laboratory values are obtained:

> Serum electrolytes (mEq/L): Na^+ 127; K^+ 5.9; Cl^- 92; HCO_3^- 15
> Blood urea nitrogen: 82 mg/100 ml
> Serum creatinine: 6.7 mg/100 ml

The patient has gained 4 kg since surgery and is mildly dyspneic at rest. Eight hours after the above data are reported, the electrocardiogram shown below is obtained. The initial treatment for this patient should include intravenous administration of

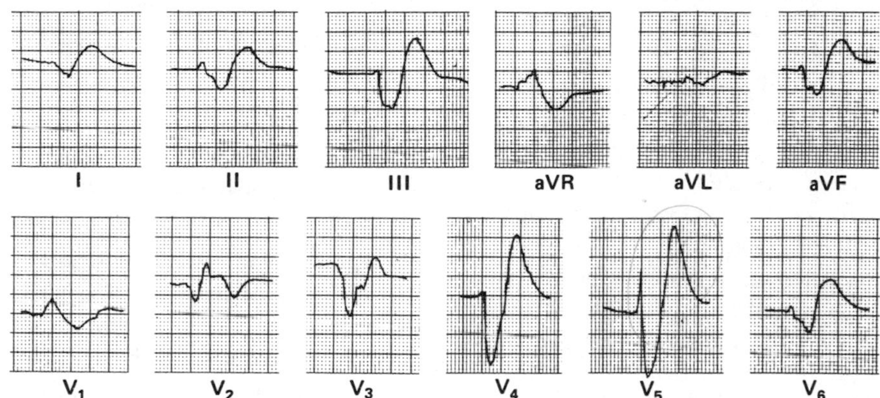

(1) 10% calcium gluconate, 10 ml
(2) digoxin, 0.25 mg every 3 hr for three doses
(3) sodium bicarbonate, 44 mEq (50 ml)
(4) lidocaine, 100 mg

SUMMARY OF DIRECTIONS

A	B	C	D	E
1,2,3 only	1,3 only	2,4 only	4 only	All are correct

24. Correct statements concerning the role of magnesium in body chemistry include which of the following?

(1) Magnesium deficiency is characterized by generalized neuromuscular hyperactivity
(2) Renal mechanisms to conserve magnesium are relatively efficient
(3) Magnesium deficiency may occur in the setting of protracted gastrointestinal losses, acute pancreatitis, and burns
(4) Magnesium toxicity may be precipitated by commonly given antacids and laxatives

25. A 68-year-old man comes to the emergency room complaining of inability to void. Physical examination reveals a distended bladder and an enlarged prostate. A Foley catheter is inserted into his bladder and 875 ml of urine are obtained. During the next hour an additional 600 ml are produced with the catheter still in place. Further management of the patient should involve

(1) matching the urine flow with intravenous 5% dextrose solution to prevent dehydration
(2) administering intravenous 0.45% NaCl while waiting for urine [Na^+] and [K^+] determinations
(3) administering 5 U vasopressin
(4) admitting the patient to the hospital

26. Four days after surgical evacuation of an acute subdural hematoma, a 44-year-old man becomes mildly lethargic and develops asterixis. He has received 2400 ml of 5% dextrose in water intravenously each day since surgery, and he appears well hydrated. Pertinent laboratory values are as follows:

Serum electrolytes (mEq/L): Na^+ 118; K^+ 3.4; Cl^- 82; HCO_3^- 24
Serum osmolality: 242 mOsm/L
Urine sodium: 47 mEq/L
Urine osmolality: 486 mOsm/L

Correct statements about this patient's fluid and electrolyte status include which of the following?

(1) His low serum sodium indicates sodium deficiency, which should be treated with 3% saline infusion
(2) He probably has the syndrome of inappropriate secretion of antidiuretic hormone
(3) His blood glucose level should be checked since the hyponatremia may be artifactual
(4) Water restriction is the cornerstone of therapy

27. Increased intracranial pressure may be treated by which of the following measures?

(1) Hyperventilation
(2) Administration of steroids
(3) Surgical decompression
(4) Administration of hypotonic solutions

28. Hypocalcemia is associated with

(1) alkalosis
(2) prolonged Q-T interval
(3) hypomagnesemia
(4) myocardial depression

29. Enteric fluids having electrolyte (Na^+, K^+, Cl^-) contents similar to Ringer's lactate include

(1) saliva
(2) ileal contents
(3) right colon contents
(4) bile

30. Sodium polystyrene sulfonate (Kayexalate) therapy can involve which of the following complications?

(1) Congestive heart failure
(2) Hyperkalemia
(3) Fecal impaction
(4) Acidosis

Questions 31–32

The two solutions most commonly used to maintain fluid and electrolyte balance in the postoperative management of patients are 5% dextrose in 0.9% sodium chloride, and lactated Ringer's solution.

31. Correct statements regarding 5% dextrose in 0.9% saline include which of the following?

(1) It contains the same concentration of sodium ions as does plasma
(2) It can be given in large quantities without seriously affecting acid-base balance
(3) It is isosmotic with plasma
(4) It has a pH of less than 7.0

32. Correct statements regarding lactated Ringer's solution include which of the following?

(1) It contains the same concentration of sodium ions as does plasma
(2) It can be given in large quantities without seriously affecting acid-base balance
(3) It is isosmotic with plasma
(4) It has a pH of less than 7.0

DIRECTIONS: Each group of questions below consists of lettered headings followed by a set of numbered items. For each numbered item select the **one** lettered heading with which it is **most** closely associated. Each lettered heading may be used **once, more than once, or not at all.**

Questions 33–36

A 42-year-old man has a calculated resting energy expenditure of 1800 kcal/day (basal energy expenditure plus 10 percent). Match the following clinical situations with the appropriate daily energy requirement.

(A) 1600
(B) 2300
(C) 2800
(D) 3600
(E) 4500

33. Sepsis

34. Skeletal trauma

35. Third degree burns of 60 percent of body surface area (BSA)

36. Prolonged starvation

Questions 37–40

Match the gastrointestinal content at each site with its appropriate ionic composition (mEq/L).

	Na	K	C1	HCO_3
(A)	140	5	104	30
(B)	140	5	75	115
(C)	60	10	130	0
(D)	10	26	10	30
(E)	60	30	40	50

37. Salivary

38. Stomach

39. Small Bowel

40. Colon

Pre- and Postoperative Care Answers

1. The answer is A. *(Schwartz, ed 5. pp 81–82.)* States of magnesium excess are characterized by generalized neuromuscular depression. Clinically, severe hypermagnesemia is rarely seen except in those patients with advanced renal failure treated with magnesium-containing antacids. Hypermagnesemia is produced intentionally, however, by those obstetricians using parenteral magnesium sulfate ($MgSO_4$) to treat preeclampsia. $MgSO_4$ is administered until depression of the deep tendon reflexes is observed, a deficit that occurs with modest hypermagnesemia (over 4 mEq/L). Greater elevations of magnesium produce progressive weakness, culminating in flaccid quadriplegia and in some cases respiratory arrest from paralysis of the chest bellows mechanism. Hypotension may occur because of the direct arteriolar relaxing effect of magnesium. Changes in mental status occur in the late stages of the syndrome and are characterized by somnolence that progresses to coma.

2. The answer is B. *(Braunwald, ed 11. pp 200–203.)* Diuretic abuse, cirrhosis, and nephrosis, by impairing the kidney's ability to dilute the urine, all produce hyponatremia. Adrenal insufficiency leads to loss of sodium (mineralocorticoid insufficiency) and an inability to excrete water (glucocorticoid deficiency), which combine to produce hyponatremia. In diabetes insipidus, the kidney is unable to conserve water, and hypernatremia develops unless antidiuretic hormone is administered or massive water intake is maintained.

3. The answer is A. *(Braunwald, ed 11. pp 1881–1883.)* High-dose glucocorticoids and mithramycin both oppose mobilization of skeletal calcium and are useful in the initial treatment of hypercalcemia of any cause. The potent "loop" diuretics, such as furosemide, increase renal calcium clearance and are especially useful when combined with saline infusions to promote a natriuresis. Phosphate infusions reduce the calcium concentration by raising the calcium-phosphorus product. Unfortunately, the resultant extraskeletal deposition of calcium is potentially dangerous, and deaths have resulted from this form of therapy. Unlike furosemide, thiazide diuretics do not block the active reabsorption of calcium by the distal tubule. By inducing depletion of fluid volume and increasing proximal tubular reabsorption of all components of the glomerular filtrate, thiazide diuretics may in fact *cause* hypercalcemia; they should be avoided in the presence of hypercalcemia.

4. The answer is C. *(Schwartz, ed 5. p 82.)* Magnesium deficiency is common in malnourished patients and patients with large gastrointestinal fluid losses. The neuromuscular effects resemble those of calcium deficiency—namely, paresthesia, hyperreflexia, muscle spasm, and ultimately tetany. The cardiac effects are more like those of hypocalcemia. An electrocardiogram therefore provides a rapid means of differentiating between hypocalcemia and hypomagnesemia. Hypomagnesemia also causes potassium wasting by the kidney. Many hospital patients with refractory hypocalcemia will be found to be magnesium deficient. Often this deficiency becomes manifest during the response to parenteral nutrition when normal cellular ionic gradients are restored. A normal blood pH and arterial P_{CO_2} rule out hyperventilation. The serum calcium in this patient is normal, when adjusted for the low albumin. Hypomagnesemia causes functional hypoparathyroidism, which can lower serum calcium, resulting in a combined defect.

5. The answer is A. *(Schwartz, ed 5. p 75.)* Hypernatremia is often associated with an extracellular fluid volume deficit when the volume lost has been hypotonic. This is a condition in which dry, sticky, mucous membranes are characteristic. Decreased body temperature, decreased deep tendon reflexes, and stupor and coma are all characteristic of extracellular fluid volume deficit secondary to isotonic fluid losses.

6. The answer is E. *(Sabiston, ed 13. pp 362–367.)* Patients with renal disease are unable to excrete the usual amounts of potassium, magnesium, and phosphate. If their urine volume is low, they will also have a tendency to accumulate fluid, leading to congestive heart failure. Hyperkalemia is particularly dangerous because it depresses myocardial activity. The acidosis of renal failure compounds reduced excretion by inhibiting cellular uptake of potassium. Hypermagnesemia is almost always iatrogenic. Many antacids and cathartics contain magnesium and their use should be restricted in renal failure. Hypermagnesemia causes weakness, hypotension, and respiratory depression. These effects are used by obstetricians to suppress preeclampsia. Chronic elevation of phosphate levels is common in patients with renal failure. Reciprocal depression of calcium levels produces secondary hyperparathyroidism, which depletes bone of calcium. Renal failure also causes a reduction of vitamin D activity with a consequent fall in intestinal calcium absorption. For these reasons such patients often need increased amounts of calcium.

7. The answer is D. *(Braunwald, ed 11. pp 212–213.)* Both the arterial pH and the P_{CO_2} are elevated in the patient presented in the question; the disturbance is alkalosis with hypoventilation. The P_{CO_2} typically increases by 0.5 to 1.0 torr for each mEq/L increase in serum bicarbonate. These findings suggest that the hypoventilation is compensatory rather than a primary phenomenon. This assumption is further supported by the absence of clinical lung disease.

8. The answer is A. *(Braunwald, ed 11. pp 212–213. Seldin, Kidney Int 1:306, 1972.)* The development of a clinically significant metabolic alkalosis in a patient requires not only the loss of acid or addition of alkali, but renal responses that *maintain* the alkalosis. The normal kidney can tremendously augment its excretion of acid or alkali in response to changes in ingested load. However, in the presence of significant volume depletion and consequent avid salt and water retention, the tubular maximum for bicarbonate reabsorption is increased. Correction of volume depletion alone is usually sufficient to correct the alkalosis, since the kidney will then excrete the excess bicarbonate. HCl infusion is usually unnecessary and can be dangerous. Acetazolamide is unlikely to be effective in the face of distal Na^+ reabsorption (in exchange for H^+ secretion). Moreover, to the extent that acetazolamide causes natriuresis, it will exacerbate the volume depletion.

9. The answer is C. *(Braunwald, ed 11. pp 1724–1729.)* Diabetes insipidus, either transient or permanent, may follow trauma to the central nervous system, especially basilar skull fractures (as in the patient presented in the question) or surgery in the area of the hypothalamic-pituitary axis. Water losses may be dramatic, with urine volumes of 30 L/24 hr. Management confined to observation, therefore, is ill-advised. Attempts to match urine output with dextrose infusions are needlessly hazardous in view of the more specific therapy available. Saline infusions are inappropriate because they also aggravate the existent water diuresis. Affected patients should receive 2 to 5 U aqueous arginine vasopressin, which has a duration of action of a few hours. For the patients who develop permanent diabetes insipidus, vasopressin tannate in oil becomes the preferred treatment because of its 2-to-3-day duration of action. This duration makes the drug undesirable for patients whose polyuria may be short-lived and might be followed by a phase of antidiuresis.

10. The answer is D. *(Emmet, Medicine 56:38–54, 1978.)* The patient presented in the question is in a state of metabolic acidosis as demonstrated by a markedly increased anion gap of 28 mEq unmeasured anions per liter of plasma. However, the respiratory response is greater than can be explained by a compensatory response, since the patient is mildly alkalemic. The disturbance cannot be a pure respiratory alkalosis, since the serum bicarbonate does not drop below 15 mEq/L as a result of renal compensation, and the anion gap does not vary more than 1 to 2 mEq/L from its normal value of 12 in response to a respiratory disturbance. The renal response to hyperventilation involves wasting of bicarbonate and compensatory retention of chloride; it does not involve a change in the concentration of ''unmeasured'' anions.

11. The answer is B. *(Anderson, Ann Intern Med 85:745–748, 1976. Braunwald, ed 11. pp 848–849.)* The acid-base disturbance in the patient described in the previous question demonstrates the value of extracting all available information from a small amount of rapidly retrievable data—e.g., arterial blood gases. Salicylates directly stimulate the respiratory center, producing respiratory alkalosis. By building up an accumulation of organic acids, salicylates also produce a concomitant metabolic acidosis. Characteristically both disturbances exist simultaneously following massive ingestion of salicylates. If sedative agents have been taken as well, the respiratory alkalosis (and even the respiratory compensation) may be absent. Phenformin and methanol overdoses also produce ''high anion-gap'' metabolic acidosis, but without the simultaneous respiratory disturbance. In the case presented, the patient's history of tinnitus in conjunction with her mixed metabolic acidosis–respiratory alkalosis is essentially pathognomonic of salicylate intoxication.

12. The answer is D. *(Fischer, pp 668, 686.)* Deficiencies of essential fatty acids, chromium, magnesium, and zinc may all develop in patients on long-term TPN. Dermatitis, alopecia, and poor wound healing along with disorders in taste are characteristic of zinc deficiency. Zinc deficiency develops more commonly in patients with gastrointestinal disease, especially diarrhea. Essential fatty acid deficiency is characterized by dry, flaky skin and hair loss. It is rarely seen now that lipid emulsions are widely used in clinical practice. Chromium deficiency often presents as the development of a diabetic state and peripheral neuropathy. The new onset of glucose intolerance should not be confused with catheter sepsis, which often presents initially as glucose intolerance. Magnesium deficiency presents with a neuromuscular syndrome similar to that of hypocalcemia and includes muscle tremors, hyperactive deep tendon reflexes, tetany, and positive Chvostek's sign.

13. The answer is C. *(Schwartz, ed 5. pp 1504–1507.)* Acute mesenteric ischemia may be difficult to diagnose. The condition should be suspected in patients with either systemic manifestations of arteriosclerotic vascular disease or low cardiac output states associated with a sudden development of abdominal pain that is out of proportion to the physical findings. Lactic acidosis and an elevated hematocrit reflecting hemoconcentration are common laboratory findings. Abdominal films show a nonspecific ileus pattern. The cause may be embolization of thrombosis of the superior mesenteric artery, primary mesenteric venous occlusion, or nonocclusive mesenteric ischemia secondary to low cardiac output states. A mortality of 65 to 100 percent is reported. The majority of affected patients are high operative risks, but since early diagnosis followed by revascularization or resectional surgery or both is the only hope for survival, celiotomy must be performed once the diagnosis of arterial occlusion or bowel infarction has been made. Initial treatment of nonocclusive mesenteric ischemia includes measures to increase cardiac output and blood pressure and the direct intraarterial superior mesenteric infusion of vasodilators such as papaverine. The patient presented in the question is at risk for both occlusive and nonocclusive mesenteric ischemic disease. If his clinical status permits, angiographic studies should be performed before the operation to establish the diagnosis and to determine whether embolectomy, revascularization, or nonsurgical management is indicated as initial treatment.

14. The answer is A. *(Sabiston, ed 13. p 95.)* The work of Goldman and others has served to identify risk factors for perioperative myocardial infarction. The highest likelihood is associated with recent myocardial infarction: the more recent the event the higher the risk up to 6 months. It should be noted, however, that the risk never returns to normal. A non–Q-wave infarction may not have destroyed much myocardium, but it leaves the surrounding area with borderline perfusion, hence the particularly high risk for subsequent perioperative infarction. Evidence of congestive heart failure, such as jugular venous distention, or S3 gallop also carries a high risk, as does the frequent occurrence of ectopic beats. Old age and emergency surgery are risk factors independent of these others. Coronary revascularization by coronary artery bypass graft (CABG) tends to protect against myocardial infarction. Smoking, diabetes, hypertension, and hyperlipidemia (all of which predispose to coronary artery disease) are surprisingly not independent risk factors, although they may increase the death rate should an infarct occur. The value of this information and data derived from further testing is that it identifies the patient who needs to be monitored invasively with a systemic arterial catheter and pulmonary arterial catheter. Most perioperative infarcts occur postoperatively when the ''third-space'' fluids return to the circulation, increasing the preload and increasing the myocardial oxygen consumption. This generally occurs around the third postoperative day.

15. The answer is A. *(Schwartz, ed 5. p 113.)* Von Willebrand's disease has an autosomal dominant pattern of inheritance affecting both men and women. The deficiency of factor VIII activity is generally less severe than in classic hemophilia and tends to fluctuate even in an untreated patient. However, the bleeding tendency is compounded by abnormal platelet function. This is responsible for the common occurrence of epistaxis and menorrhagia. In 70 percent of patients platelets fail to aggregate in response to ristocetin. Transfusion of cryoprecipitate provides factor VIII R:WF (the von Willebrand factor), whereas infusions of high-purity concentrates of factor VIII:C are not effective. These patients do not generally require treatment unless they need surgery or are severely injured; therefore, they have not usually received the contaminated concentrates responsible for the 80 percent prevalence of HIV seropositivity among hemophiliacs.

16. The answer is B. *(Sabiston, ed 13. pp 1719–1721.)* This patient has a left ileofemoral vein thrombosis, as evidenced by sudden massive swelling of her entire left lower extremity. Noninvasive venous testing should be quite helpful as the venous obstruction extends above the knee and therefore venography and x-ray exposure are unnecessary. Heparin is the preferred agent because it does not cross the placenta. The vena caval filter is not indicated because there is no contraindication to heparin therapy and there has not been any evidence of pulmonary embolus.

17. The answer is B. *(Schwartz, ed 5. pp 117–118.)* Intraoperative and postoperative hemorrhage is a significant problem in the patient with polycythemia vera.

Despite thrombocytosis, these patients have a hemorrhagic tendency generally ascribed to a qualitative deficiency of the platelets. Elective surgery should be postponed until the hematocrit and platelet count reach normal levels. Alkylating agents, such as busulfan or chlorambucil, are effective in this regard. In the emergency situation, phlebectomy should be performed prior to operation and especially careful hemostatic technique should be employed. Infection also is a problem in patients with polycythemia vera, but hemorrhagic problems are the more frequently encountered complications.

18. The answer is C. *(Schwartz, ed 5. p 130.)* When large amounts of banked blood are transfused, the recipient becomes deficient in factors V and VIII (the "labile" factors) and an acquired coagulopathy ensues. Since banked blood is also deficient in platelets, thrombocytopenia may also develop.

19. The answer is C. *(Sabiston, ed 13. pp 558–561.)* The superior laryngeal nerve courses near the superior thyroid artery and may be injured during thyroidectomy. The nerve innervates the cricothyroid muscle but has no effect on the true vocal cords themselves. Injury to the nerve produces no immediate voice change; with prolonged use the voice loses its timbre. Injury to the recurrent laryngeal nerve causes instantaneous dysphonia. Thyroid surgery occasionally is followed by other important complications. The thyroid gland is highly vascular and postoperative hemorrhage may occur following any thyroid surgery. The parathyroids are sometimes inadvertently removed or damaged and prolonged derangement in calcium metabolism may occur.

20. The answer is A (1, 2, 3). *(Schwartz, ed 5. p 80.)* Reduction of an elevated serum potassium level is important to avoid the cardiovascular complications that ultimately culminate in diastolic cardiac arrest. Kayexalate is a cation exchange resin that is instilled into the gastrointestinal tract and exchanges sodium for potassium ions. Its use is limited to semiacute and chronic potassium elevations. Sodium bicarbonate causes a rise in serum pH and shifts potassium intracellularly. Administration of glucose initiates glycogen synthesis and uptake of potassium. Insulin can be used in conjunction with this to aid in the shift of potassium intracellularly. Calcium gluconate does not affect the serum potassium level but rather counteracts the myocardial effects of hyperkalemia.

21. The answer is B (1, 3). *(Schwartz, ed 5. p 81.)* Postthyroidectomy hypocalcemia is usually due to transient ischemia of the parathyroid glands and is self-limited. When it becomes symptomatic it should be treated with intravenous infusions of calcium. In most cases the problem is resolved in several days. If hypocalcemia persists, oral therapy is started with calcium gluconate. Vitamin D preparations are only used if hypocalcemia is prolonged and permanent hypoparathyroidism is suspected.

22. The answer is B (1, 3). *(Schwartz, ed 5. p 100.)* Vitamin K and folic acid are both unstable in solution and cannot be infused with TPN solutions. Prothrombin times should be checked weekly and vitamin K administered intramuscularly as needed. Folic acid should be administered intramuscularly weekly to prevent deficiencies from developing.

23. The answer is B (1, 3). *(Braunwald, ed 11. pp 207–208, 880.)* The electrocardiogram exhibited in the question demonstrates changes that are essentially diagnostic of severe hyperkalemia. Correct treatment for the affected patient includes administration of a source of calcium ions (which will immediately oppose the neuromuscular effect of potassium) and administration of sodium ions (which, by producing a mild alkalosis, will shift potassium into cells); each will temporarily reduce serum potassium concentration. Infusion of glucose and insulin would also effect a temporary transcellular shift of potassium. However, these maneuvers are only temporarily effective; definitive treatment calls for removal of potassium from the body. The sodium-potassium exchange resin sodium polystyrene sulfonate (Kayexalate) would accomplish this removal but at the price of adding a sodium ion for each potassium ion that is removed. Hemodialysis or peritoneal dialysis is probably required for this patient, since these procedures also rectify the other consequences of acute renal failure. Both lidocaine and digoxin would not only be ineffective but contraindicated, since they would further depress the myocardial conduction system.

24. The answer is E (all). *(Schwartz, ed 5. pp 81–82.)* Along with potassium and calcium, magnesium is very important in the regulation of many enzyme systems in the body. The clinical manifestations of disturbances of magnesium levels are primarily related to the neuromuscular (including cardiac) functions and the central nervous system. Magnesium deficiency tends to mimic calcium deficiency, with which it often coexists. Patients who are receiving total parenteral nutrition need to be watched carefully for magnesium deficiency. Magnesium deficiency may be rapidly corrected (if clinically indicated) by the intravenous infusion of magnesium chloride or sulfate, but one must be careful not to overshoot. The kidneys are very effective and important in regulating serum levels of magnesium and ordinarily are quite good at conserving magnesium. Renal excretion depends on glomerular and tubular function. In patients with renal failure it is quite possible to achieve toxic levels of magnesium even with ordinary dosages of magnesium-containing antacids and cathartics. Some of the more widely used magnesium-containing agents are Maalox and Gelusil. Magnesium toxicity involves CNS depression and muscle weakness with depression of deep tendon reflexes. The ECG changes seen resemble those produced by excess potassium. Acute management may include intravenous calcium chloride or gluconate.

25. The answer is C (2, 4). *(Braunwald, ed 11. p 1218.)* Postobstructive diuresis is frequently observed but poorly understood; it occurs clinically only after relief of bilateral obstruction. In this condition, urine flow may approach 50 percent of the glomerular filtration rate. Frequently, the polyuria is physiologic (as in the excretion of retained salt and water), but it can be iatrogenic (as in the diuresis maintained by overly vigorous administration of intravenous fluids). If azotemia has developed, the excretion of the retained urea may maintain an osmotic diuresis. In some cases, obstruction can produce intrinsic tubular defects in sodium reabsorption resulting in urinary concentration; in these cases, the pathologic salt and water losses must be replaced. Proper management of the postobstructive patient includes frequent clinical assessment of the patient's fluid volume status (physical examination, intake and output measurements, frequent weight determinations) and electrolyte balance, coupled with replacement of excess salt and water losses. Intravenous glucose alone is inappropriate because it may induce an osmotic diuresis while failing to replace urinary sodium, potassium, and chloride losses. Vasopressin administration is ineffective in the presence of a tubular defect in urinary concentration.

26. The answer is C (2, 4). *(Schwartz, ed 5. pp 24, 56.)* The findings in the patient presented in the question are typical of the syndrome of inappropriate antidiuretic hormone secretion (SIADH). Although this syndrome is primarily associated with diseases of the central nervous system or of the chest (e.g., oat cell carcinoma of the lung), excessive amounts of antidiuretic hormone are also present in most postoperative patients. The pathophysiology of SIADH involves an inability to dilute the urine, and administered water is therefore retained, producing dilutional hyponatremia. Body sodium stores and fluid balance are normal, as evidenced by the absence of the clinical findings suggestive of abnormalities of extracellular fluid volume. While hypertonic saline infusions can transiently improve hyponatremia, the appropriate therapy is to restrict water ingestion to a level below the patient's ability to excrete water. Hypertonic saline may be dangerous, since it can shift accumulated water into the extracellular fluid and precipitate pulmonary edema in the patient who suffers from low cardiac reserves. Hyperglycemia cannot account for the hyponatremia seen in this patient, because the serum osmolality, as well as the serum sodium, is depressed. Hyponatremia resulting from hyperglycemia would be associated with an elevated serum osmolality.

27. The answer is A (1, 2, 3). *(Sabiston, ed 13. p 1383.)* The cerebrovascular bed volume is dependent upon arterial pressure, venous pressure, and the CO_2 content of the circulating blood. Because hypoxia and hypercapnia significantly increase intracranial pressure, hyperventilation can be lifesaving in patients who have acute intracranial hypertension. Arterial pressure should not be reduced, but the venous pressure should be kept as low as possible by slight elevation of the head, by keeping the intravascular volume as low as possible, by avoiding airway obstruction, and by avoiding prolonged positive pressure respiratory cycles. The administration of steroids also seems to reduce brain edema, probably by altering cell membrane function. Surgical decompression, although it allows the edema to form, may reduce the likelihood of a fatal brainstem herniation. Some workers have recommended hypertonic solutions to reduce edema associated with increased intracranial pressure; hypotonic solutions may increase edema and should be avoided.

28. The answer is E (all). *(Braunwald, ed 11. p 89. Schwartz, ed 5. p 81.)* Hypocalcemia is associated with a prolonged Q-T interval and may be aggravated by both hypomagnesemia and alkalosis. Serum calcium levels below 7.0 mg/dl, encountered most frequently following parathyroid or thyroid surgery, or in patients with acute pancreatitis, should be treated with intravenous calcium gluconate or lactate. The myocardium is very sensitive to calcium levels; therefore calcium is considered a positive inotropic agent. Calcium increases the contractile strength of cardiac muscle as well as the velocity of shortening. In its absence the efficiency of the myocardium decreases.

29. The answer is C (2, 4). *(Schwartz, ed 5. pp 73, 83.)* Bile and the fluids found in the duodenum, jejunum, and ileum all have electrolyte contents similar to Ringer's lactate. Saliva and right colon fluids have high potassium and low Na^+ content. It is important to consider these variations in electrolyte patterns when calculating replacement requirements following gastrointestinal losses.

30. The answer is B (1, 3). *(Braunwald, ed 11. pp 208, 1154. Townsend, N Engl J Med 288:1058, 1973.)* Sodium polystyrene sulfonate, a nonabsorbable sodium-potassium exchange resin, is useful in the management of moderate-to-severe hyperkalemia. Each gram of resin will remove approximately 1 mEq potassium from the body. However, the resin also binds H^+ ions, and for each mEq of K^+ removed, roughly 2 mEq of Na^+ are added to the body stores. The resultant fluid retention can limit the utility of this resin in the oliguric patient who is unable to withstand further expansion of extracellular fluid volume. Compaction of resin in the colon produced by absorption of water from intestinal contents results in fecal impaction. This problem can be averted by mixing the resin in a slurry of 25 to 75% sorbitol to promote osmotic diarrhea.

31–32. The answers are: 31-D (4), 32-C (2, 4). *(Schwartz, ed 5. p 83.)* Isotonic saline solutions contain 154 mEq/L of both sodium and chloride ions. Each ion is in a substantially higher concentration than is found in the normal serum (Na = 142 mEq/L; Cl = 103 mEq/L). When isotonic solutions are given in large quantities, they overload the kidney's ability to excrete chloride ion, which results in a dilutional acidosis. They also may intensify preexisting acidosis by reducing the base bicarbonate/carbonic acid ratio in the body. Isotonic saline solutions are particularly useful in hyponatremic or hypochloremic states and whenever a tendency to metabolic alkalosis is present, as occurs with significant nasogastric suction losses or vomiting.

Administration of lactated Ringer's solution is appropriate for replacing gastrointestinal losses and correcting extracellular fluid deficits. Containing 130 mEq/L sodium, lactated Ringer's is hyposmolar with respect to sodium and provides approximately 150 ml of free water with each liter given. Although ordinarily not a significant load, in some clinical situations it can be. Lactated Ringer's is sufficiently "physiological" to enable administration of large amounts without affecting the body's acid-base balance significantly. It is worth noting that both isotonic saline and lactated Ringer's are acid with respect to the plasma: 0.9% NaCl / 5% dextrose has a pH of 4.5; lactated Ringer's has a pH of 6.5.

33–36. The answers are: 33-C, 34-B, 35-D, 36-A. *(Elwyn, p 550.)* Resting energy expenditure in the nonstressed patient is approximately 10 percent greater than basal energy expenditure. The resting energy expenditure increases directly proportional to the degree of stress. Studies by Kinney and associates using indirect calorimetry have documented the relative degree of increase in resting energy expenditure for a variety of clinical situations. The following table summarizes these results.

Clinical Situation	Change in Energy Expenditure
Prolonged starvation	Decreased 10–30%
Skeletal trauma	Increased 10–30%
Sepsis	Increased 30–60%
3rd degree burns over greater than 20% BSA	Increased 50–100%

37–40. The answers are: 37-D, 38-C, 39-A, 40-E. *(Schwartz, ed 5. p 73.)* One of the commonest causes of dehydration and metabolic disarray in surgical patients is the failure to replace gastrointestinal losses. External losses can often be collected for measurement of volume and ionic composition. Accurate replacement of these measured losses is clearly the best method of avoiding imbalance. However, a knowledge of the ionic composition of the intestinal contents at various sites permits an accurate estimate for early replacement. Most of these secretions start as extracellular fluid (with a composition similar to that of plasma) and are modified by intestinal glands. The stomach substitutes hydrogen ions for sodium, thus eliminating all but a tiny fraction of bicarbonate. The glands of the small intestine secrete various amounts of bicarbonate; the chloride content is depressed to an equivalent degree (to maintain ionic balance). Colonic contents (stool) and saliva are most notable for their potassium content. Stool also has a high bicarbonate content. Severe diarrhea can therefore cause potassium depletion and a metabolic acidosis.

Critical Care: Anesthesiology, Blood Gases, Respiratory Care

DIRECTIONS: Each question below contains five suggested responses. Select the **one best** response to each question.

41. The consequences of hyperbaric spinal anesthesia include all the following physiologic responses EXCEPT

(A) increased gastrointestinal motility
(B) adequate sensory anesthesia
(C) respiratory paralysis
(D) venous dilatation
(E) headache

42. All the following statements concerning local anesthetics are true EXCEPT

(A) bupivacaine (Marcaine) is particularly likely to cause a cardiac arrest after inadvertent intravenous injection
(B) use of epinephrine increases the dose of lidocaine that can be given safely
(C) intercostal blockade is associated with rapid absorption of local anesthetics
(D) lidocaine may be given in doses up to 6 mg/kg over a 15 minute period
(E) intravenous lidocaine can be used to suppress the cough reflex during endotracheal suctioning

43. Hyperventilation alleviates the symptoms of increased intracranial pressure as a result of which of the following mechanisms?

(A) Improved cerebral oxygen delivery
(B) Reduced ionized calcium concentration, which raises the seizure threshold
(C) Decreased cerebral blood flow, which reduces intracranial filtration pressure
(D) Induced respiratory alkalosis, which counteracts the cerebral lactic acidosis
(E) None of the above

44. The partial pressure of halothane in arterial blood rises more rapidly when halothane is administered with nitrous oxide (N_2O) than when halothane is administered alone. This effect can be attributed to the

(A) respiratory stimulant effect of N_2O
(B) solubility of halothane in N_2O
(C) reduced blood : gas partition coefficient for halothane
(D) N_2-N_2O blood solubility differences
(E) fact that displaced alveolar air is heavier than the combined anesthetic gas mixture

45. In a hemolytic reaction caused by an incompatible blood transfusion, the treatment that is LEAST likely to be helpful is

(A) promoting a diuresis with 20 percent mannitol
(B) preventing anuria through fluid and potassium replacement
(C) alkalinizing the urine with sodium bicarbonate
(D) inserting a Foley catheter to monitor hourly urine output
(E) stopping the blood transfusion immediately

46. The concept of minimum alveolar anesthetic concentration (MAC) represents an important advance in the understanding and use of inhalation anesthetics. All the following statements regarding MAC are true EXCEPT that

(A) MAC is defined as the alveolar concentration of an anesthetic that prevents response to pain in 50 percent of subjects
(B) nitrous oxide increases the MAC of halothane
(C) alveolar partial pressures closely reflect the anesthetic partial pressures in arterial blood and the central nervous system
(D) MAC is a reference standard for comparing toxicity of inhalation anesthetics
(E) MAC refers to alveolar, not inspired, concentration of anesthetic

47. A 64-year-old man afflicted with severe emphysema, who receives oxygen therapy at home, is admitted to the hospital because of upper gastrointestinal bleeding. The bleeding ceases soon after admission, and the patient becomes agitated and then disoriented; he is given intramuscular diazepam (Valium), 5 mg. Twenty minutes later he is unresponsive. Physical examination reveals a stuporous but arousable man who has papilledema and asterixis. Arterial blood gases are pH 7.17, P_{O_2} 42 torr, P_{CO_2} 95 torr. The best immediate therapy would be to

(A) correct hypoxemia with high-flow nasal oxygen
(B) correct acidosis with sodium bicarbonate
(C) administer intravenous dexamethasone, 10 mg
(D) intubate the patient
(E) call for neurosurgical consultation

Questions 48–50

A 32-year-old man undergoes a distal pancreatectomy, splenectomy, and partial colectomy for a gunshot wound to the left upper quadrant of the abdomen. One week later he develops a shaking chill in conjunction with a temperature spike to 39.44°C (103°F). His blood pressure is 70/0 with a pulse of 140 beats/min and his respiratory rate is 45 breaths/min. He is transferred to the ICU where he is intubated and a Swan-Ganz catheter is placed.

48. Which of the following would be most consistent with this patient's preintubation arterial blood gas measurements?

	pH	P_{CO_2}	P_{O_2}
(A)	7.31	48	61
(B)	7.52	28	76
(C)	7.45	40	77
(D)	7.40	30	72
(E)	7.40	48	94

49. All the following are consistent with the initial Swan-Ganz catheter readings EXCEPT

(A) cardiac output: 9.0 L/min
(B) peripheral vascular resistance: 1660 dynes
(C) pulmonary artery pressure: 33/3 mmHg
(D) pulmonary capillary wedge pressure: 3 mmHg
(E) central venous pressure: 12 mmHg

50. Initial therapy for this patient would include all the following EXCEPT

(A) fluid replacement
(B) dopamine
(C) clindamycin
(D) laparotomy
(E) gentamicin

51. The most common physiologic cause of hypoxemia is

(A) hypoventilation
(B) incomplete alveolar oxygen diffusion
(C) ventilation-perfusion inequality
(D) pulmonary shunt flow
(E) elevated erythrocyte 2,3 diphosphoglycerate level (2,3 DPG)

52. The curve depicted below plots the normal relationship of arterial P_{O_2} and percentage of hemoglobin saturation with other variables controlled at pH 7.4, P_{CO_2} 40 torr, temperature 37°C (98.6°F), and hemoglobin 15 g/100 ml. All the following statements regarding this oxygen dissociation relationship are true EXCEPT that

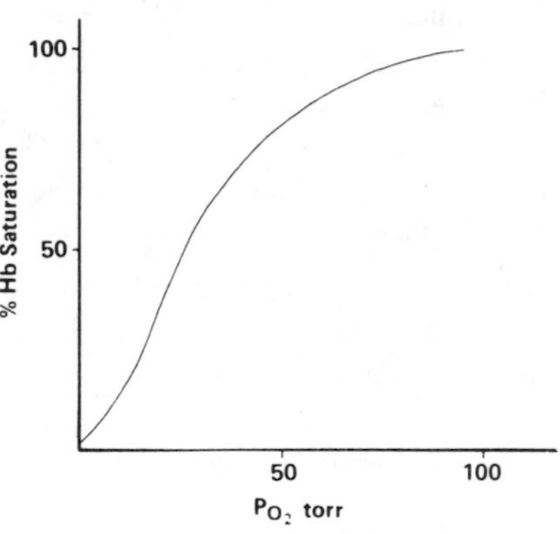

(A) modest decrements of arterial P_{O_2} have little effect on alveolar oxygen uptake
(B) modest decrements of hemoglobin saturation have little effect on tissue oxygen uptake
(C) the curve shifts to the right with acidosis
(D) the curve shifts to the left following banked blood transfusion
(E) the curve is unaffected by chronic lung disease

53. Generally accepted indications calling for mechanical ventilatory support include all the following EXCEPT

(A) P_{O_2} of less than 60 torr and P_{CO_2} of greater than 60 torr while breathing room air
(B) alveolar-arterial oxygen tension difference of 350 torr while breathing 100% O_2
(C) vital capacity of 40 to 60 ml/kg
(D) respiratory rate greater than 35/min
(E) V_D/V_T greater than 0.6

54. Which of the following inhalation anesthetics accumulates in air-filled cavities during general anesthesia?

(A) Diethyl ether
(B) Nitrous oxide
(C) Halothane
(D) Methoxyflurane
(E) Trichloroethylene

55. Improvement of tissue oxygenation in traumatized patients is best attained by the infusion of

(A) oxygenated fluorocarbon fluid
(B) bicarbonate solution
(C) frozen erythrocytes
(D) free hemoglobin
(E) free myoglobin

56. Major alterations in pulmonary function associated with adult respiratory distress syndrome (ARDS) include all the following EXCEPT

(A) hypoxemia
(B) decreased pulmonary compliance
(C) diffuse interstitial pattern on x-ray
(D) increased functional residual capacity
(E) increased dead space ventilation

57. Swan-Ganz catheterization of the pulmonary artery allows for direct measurement of all the following cardiopulmonary hemodynamics EXCEPT

(A) mixed venous oxygen saturation
(B) central venous pressure
(C) left ventricular end-diastolic pressure
(D) pulmonary vascular resistance
(E) cardiac output

58. The administration of local anesthetics may result in all the following EXCEPT

(A) tachycardia
(B) vasodilatation
(C) myocardial depression
(D) seizures
(E) failure of anesthesia in acidotic tissues

Questions 59–60

A 68-year-old hypertensive man underwent successful repair of a ruptured abdominal aortic aneurysm. He received 9 L Ringer's lactate solution and 4 units of whole blood during the operation. Two hours after transfer to the surgical intensive care unit the following hemodynamic parameters are obtained:

Systemic blood pressure (BP): 90/60 mmHg
Pulse rate: 110/min
Central venous pressure (CVP): 7 mmHg
Pulmonary artery pressure: 28/10
Pulmonary capillary wedge pressure: 8 mmHg
Cardiac output: 1.9 L/min
Systemic vascular resistance: 35 Woods units (normal 24 to 30 Woods units)
Pa_{O_2}: 140 torr (FI_{O_2} .45)
Urine output: 15 ml/hr (specific gravity 1.029)
Hematocrit: 35%

59. Proper management would now call for

(A) administration of a diuretic to increase urine output
(B) administration of a vasopressor agent to increase the systemic blood pressure
(C) administration of a fluid challenge to increase the urine output
(D) administration of a vasodilating agent to decrease the elevated systemic vascular resistance
(E) a period of observation to obtain more data

60. The patient then does well with an improvement in all hemodynamic parameters. However, 6 hr later he develops inverted T waves and diffuse ST-T wave changes on his ECG. New hemodynamic parameters are obtained:

Systemic BP: 60/40 mmHg
Pulse rate: 120/min
CVP: 13 mmHg
Pulmonary capillary wedge pressure: 22 mmHg
Cardiac output: 1.5 L/min

Management would now include

(A) administration of an inotropic agent
(B) administration of a vasopressor agent
(C) administration of a fluid challenge
(D) operative reexploration
(E) emergency angiogram

61. A 56-year-old man undergoes a left upper lobectomy. An epidural catheter is inserted for postoperative pain relief. Ninety minutes after the first dose of epidural morphine the patient complains of itching and is becoming increasingly somnolent. Blood gas measurement reveals the following: pH 7.24, P_{CO_2} 58, P_{O_2} 100, and HCO_3^- 28. Initial therapy should include

(A) endotracheal intubation
(B) intramuscular diphenhydramine (Benadryl)
(C) epidural naloxone
(D) intravenous naloxone
(E) alternative analgesia

DIRECTIONS: Each question below contains four suggested responses of which **one or more** is correct. Select

A	if	**1, 2, and 3**	are correct
B	if	**1 and 3**	are correct
C	if	**2 and 4**	are correct
D	if	**4**	is correct
E	if	**1, 2, 3, and 4**	are correct

Questions 62–63

62. Malignant hyperthermia is characterized by

(1) excess calcium in myoplasm
(2) abnormal response to succinylcholine
(3) increased O_2 consumption
(4) decreased K^+

63. In patients with a history of malignant hyperthermia requiring another operation, one should

(1) pretreat with dantrolene
(2) use depolarizing muscle relaxants
(3) premedicate heavily
(4) acidify the urine

64. Noncardiac factors that can increase central venous pressure (CVP) include

(1) hypervolemia
(2) positive pressure ventilation
(3) pneumothorax
(4) flail chest

65. Signs and symptoms of unsuspected Addison's disease include

(1) hypothermia
(2) hypokalemia
(3) hyperglycemia
(4) hyponatremia

66. Correct statements concerning managing the airway in the severely traumatized patient include which of the following?

(1) Awake intubation is contraindicated in patients with penetrating ocular injuries
(2) Awake intubation or rapid sequence induction of anesthesia with intravenous thiobarbiturate followed by succinylcholine is the method of choice if intubation is deemed necessary
(3) Steroids have not been shown to be of value in the management of aspiration of acid gastric secretions
(4) Prior to endotracheal intubation, it is safe to assume that the patient's stomach is empty if a reliable history is obtained indicating that the last ingestion of food/liquid occurred 8 hr before arrival in the emergency room

SUMMARY OF DIRECTIONS

A	B	C	D	E
1,2,3 only	1,3 only	2,4 only	4 only	All are correct

67. Correct statements concerning drowning or near-drowning include which of the following?

(1) The prognosis for recovery of cerebral function in affected persons is better if submersion occurs in cool water rather than extremely cold water
(2) The presence of a significant metabolic acidosis in affected persons frequently requires the administration of intravenous sodium bicarbonate
(3) Prompt administration of corticosteroids to affected persons has been shown to decrease the extent of pulmonary membrane damage
(4) Renal damage may occur in affected persons as a result of hemoglobinuria

68. Treatment for clostridial myonecrosis (gas gangrene) includes which of the following measures?

(1) Administration of penicillin
(2) Administration of hyperbaric oxygen
(3) Wide debridement
(4) Administration of antitoxin

69. The P_{50} of normal human hemoglobin is altered by

(1) changes in arterial pH
(2) changes in tissue temperature
(3) changes in 2,3-diphosphoglycerate concentration
(4) carbon monoxide poisoning

70. A 50-year-old man about to undergo colon resection says he is unwilling to allow blood transfusion because of the risk of hepatitis. Correct statements regarding these risks include which of the following?

(1) Transfusion of two units of blood carries a 5 percent chance of hepatitis
(2) Immune serum globulin reliably prevents hepatitis B
(3) The incubation period of hepatitis B is about 2 to 3 weeks
(4) Human serum albumin infusion is rarely associated with the development of hepatitis

71. An abnormal ventilation-perfusion ratio (Qs/Qr) in the postoperative patient can result from

(1) a supine position
(2) obesity
(3) atelectasis
(4) reduced cardiac output

72. Etiologic factors implicated in the development of posttraumatic pulmonary insufficiency include

(1) increase of vasoactive substances
(2) microembolization of platelet aggregates
(3) fluid overload
(4) increased pulmonary surfactant

73. Patients with adult respiratory distress syndrome (ARDS) may benefit from the use of positive end-expiratory pressure (PEEP) because increasing expiratory threshold resistance can

(1) increase functional residual capacity
(2) increase left ventricular compliance
(3) decrease intrapulmonary shunting
(4) increase cardiac output

74. Correct statements concerning smoke inhalation ("smoke poisoning") include which of the following?

(1) "Smoke poisoning" is a chemical rather than thermal injury
(2) Carbon monoxide levels are usually elevated
(3) Chest x-rays during the early post-inhalation period are usually normal
(4) Visible damage to the respiratory tract is commonly found

75. The accidental aspiration of gastric contents into the tracheobronchial tree should be treated by

(1) tracheal suctioning
(2) bronchoscopy and lavage
(3) ventilatory support
(4) antibiotic administration to cover oral-pharyngeal anaerobes

76. In performing a tracheostomy, authorities agree that

(1) the strap muscles should be preserved and retracted
(2) the thyroid isthmus may be divided
(3) the trachea should be entered at the second or third cartilaginous ring
(4) only horizontal incisions should be used

77. Factors that increase the risk for postoperative myocardial infarction include

(1) stable angina
(2) surgery within 6 months of a prior infarction
(3) hypertension
(4) age greater than 70 years

DIRECTIONS: Each group of questions below consists of four lettered headings followed by a set of numbered items. For each numbered item select

A	if the item is associated with	(A) **only**
B	if the item is associated with	(B) **only**
C	if the item is associated with	**both** (A) and (B)
D	if the item is associated with	**neither** (A) nor (B)

Questions 78–80

(A) Curare
(B) Succinylcholine
(C) Both
(D) Neither

78. Myasthenics are quite sensitive

79. Sustained paralysis may occur

80. Hyperkalemia may be induced

Questions 81–85

(A) Normovolemic gram negative sepsis
(B) Hypovolemic gram negative sepsis
(C) Both
(D) Neither

81. Hypotension

82. High cardiac output

83. Increased peripheral vascular resistance

84. Respiratory alkalosis

85. Vasopressors in initial therapy

DIRECTIONS: Each group of questions below consists of lettered headings followed by a set of numbered items. For each numbered item select the **one** lettered heading with which it is **most** closely associated. Each lettered heading may be used **once, more than once, or not at all.**

Questions 86–89

Match the side effects below with the appropriate anesthetic.

(A) N_2O
(B) Halothane
(C) Methoxyflurane
(D) Enflurane
(E) Morphine

86. Nephrotoxicity

87. Seizures

88. Decreased peripheral resistance

89. Possible worsening of distension in bowel obstruction

Questions 90–93

Match the tests below with the coagulation system they evaluate.

(A) Intrinsic pathway
(B) Fibrinogen function
(C) Platelet function
(D) Extrinsic pathway
(E) None of the above

90. Prothrombin time

91. Bleeding time

92. Thrombin time

93. Partial thromboplastin time

Critical Care: Anesthesiology, Blood Gases, Respiratory Care

Answers

41. The answer is C. *(Schwartz, ed 5. p 464.)* The large myelinated fibers of the phrenic nerve emanating from the third through fifth cervical nerves are relatively resistant to the effects of hyperbaric spinal anesthesia. Even in the unusual circumstances when sensory anesthesia extends to the high thoracic segments, diaphragmatic function and ventilation are preserved. Local trauma at the puncture site resulting in prolonged cerebrospinal fluid leakage may lead to headaches. The incidence depends upon the size of the needle used. With larger caliber needles (18 gauge) an incidence as high as 20 percent can be expected, whereas 25 gauge needles reduce the incidence to less than 2 percent. Sympathetic blockage results in venous dilatation and uninhibited gastrointestinal motility. Because somatic sensory fibers are more easily anesthetized than large somatic motor fibers, hypoesthesia adequate to allow the skin incision may exist together with persistent muscle tone.

42. The answer is D. *(Gilman, ed 7. pp 304–305, 308, 767–770.)* Local anesthetics work by impairing the normal movement of Na^+ across the cell membranes of nerve cells. Small nonmyelinated fibers, such as those that mediate pain sensation, are most sensitive. Allergic reactions to the esters (procaine and tetracaine) do occur, but they are much less common than the toxic effects on the CNS and CVS. With increasing blood levels one sees diplopia, dizziness, confusion, seizure activity, and malignant ventricular arrhythmias such as ventricular fibrillation. The blood levels known to produce toxic reactions generally parallel the potency. One exception is the propensity for cardiac toxicity often reported with bupivacaine (Marcaine). Rates of absorption vary according to the site. The most rapid rise in blood levels follows intercostal injection. The concomitant use of epinephrine slows absorption of the anesthetic, thereby reducing the incidence of toxic reactions. In a short period of time, 6 mg/kg of lidocaine is too much to infiltrate. Paradoxically, intravenous lidocaine is used to suppress ventricular ectopy. It is also used as a prophylaxis against laryngeal spasm during the induction of anesthesia.

43. The answer is C. *(Sabiston, ed 13. p 1383.)* Cerebral blood flow remains constant over a wide range of systemic arterial pressures. When capillary injury or other vascular damage results in edema within the closed cranial cavity, the "normal" flow rate may in fact be excessive and exacerbate the edema. Reducing the arterial P_{CO_2} resets the cerebral blood flow's autoregulatory mechanisms to a lower rate of flow and thus decreases the hydrostatic forces favoring formation of edema.

44. The answer is D. *(Hardy, ed 2. pp 252–253.)* Nitrous oxide (N_2O) is 30 times more soluble in blood than is nitrogen. Hence, the uptake of nitrous oxide into the blood exceeds the excretion of N_2 from the blood. This differential between uptake and excretion leads to a transient loss of volume within the alveolus and a relative concentration of the remaining gases—oxygen, carbon dioxide, and inhaled anesthetic (i.e., halothane). This phenomenon accelerates the rate of uptake of other agents, like halothane, when they are administered with N_2O. This process is called the "second gas" effect.

45. The answer is B. *(Schwartz, ed 5. pp 131–132.)* Whenever a hemolytic reaction caused by an incompatible blood transfusion is suspected, the transfusion should be stopped immediately. A Foley catheter should be inserted, and hourly urine output should be monitored. Renal damage caused by precipitation of hemoglobin in the renal tubules is the major serious consequence of the hemolysis. This precipitation is inhibited in an alkaline environment and is promoted in an acid environment. Stimulating diuresis with 100 ml of 20 percent mannitol and alkalinizing the urine with 45 mEq sodium bicarbonate intravenously are indicated procedures. Fluid and potassium intake should be restricted in the presence of severe oliguria or anuria.

46. The answer is B. *(Schwartz, ed 5. p 462.)* The concept of MAC has proved helpful in understanding mechanisms of action of inhalation anesthetics and in the clinical use of these agents. It is defined as the alveolar concentration of an anesthetic that prevents somatic response to painful stimuli in 50 percent of subjects. Alveolar, arterial, and central nervous system partial pressures of the inhalation anesthetics are generally identical. Gradients do exist for the highly soluble anesthetics in the presence of ventilation-perfusion pulmonary abnormalities. Because anesthetic side effects are meaningful only when equieffective concentrations are compared, MAC is widely used as a reference standard for comparing different agents. Nitrous oxide is rarely used alone because of its lack of anesthetic potency. It is useful, however, in combination with more powerful agents in effecting a decrease in toxicity. Nitrous oxide, for example, decreases the MAC of halothane, permitting its use at lower concentrations and thereby decreasing its adverse side effects.

47. The answer is D. *(Schwartz, ed 5. pp 77–78.)* The patient presented in the question is suffering from acute, life-threatening respiratory acidosis that has been compounded, if not produced, by the injudicious administration of a central nervous system depressant. While hypoxemia must also be corrected, the immediate task is to correct the acidosis caused by carbon dioxide accumulation. Both disturbances can be resolved by skillful endotracheal intubation and by ventilatory support. Sodium bicarbonate and high-flow nasal oxygen would both be inappropriate. Bicarbonate should not be administered because buffer reserves already are adequate (serum bicarbonate is still 34 mEq/L based on the Henderson-Hasselbalch equation). Nasal oxygen administration is not warranted because both acidemia and hypoxemia are themselves potent stimulants to spontaneous ventilation. Headache, confusion, and papilledema all are signs of acute carbon dioxide retention and do not imply the presence of a structural intracranial lesion.

48–50. The answers are: 48-B, 49-B, 50-D. *(Schwartz, ed 5. pp 173–177.)* The case presented is most consistent with septic shock from a postoperative intraabdominal abscess. In the early phase of septic shock the respiratory profile is characterized by mild hypoxia with a compensatory hyperventilation and respiratory alkalosis. Hemodynamically a hyperdynamic state is seen with an increase in cardiac output and a decrease in peripheral vascular resistance in the face of relatively normal central pressures. Initial therapy is aimed at resuscitation and stabilization. This includes fluid replacement and vasopressors as well as antibiotic therapy aimed particularly at gram negative rods and anaerobes for patients with presumed intraabdominal collections, especially after bowel surgery. Laparotomy and drainage of a collection is the definitive therapy but should await stabilization of the patient and confirmation of the presence and location of such a collection.

51. The answer is C. *(West, ed 3. pp 49–64.)* Although hypoventilation, incomplete oxygen diffusion, and pulmonary shunts all are causes of hypoxemia, the most common cause is ventilation-perfusion inequality. The mismatch of ventilation and blood flow occurs to some degree in the normal upright lung but may become extreme in the diseased lung. The three indices used to measure ventilation-perfusion inequality are alveolar-arterial P_{O_2} difference, physiologic shunt (venous admixture), and alveolar dead space. Elevated 2,3 diphosphoglycerate (DPG) levels shift the oxygen dissociation curve to the right, thereby augmenting tissue oxygenation. This elevation does not result in hypoxemia.

52. The answer is E. *(West, ed 3. pp 69–72.)* The shape of the oxygen dissociation curve translates into several physiologic advantages. The relatively flat slope above a P_{O_2} of 50 torr means that, in this region of the curve, hemoglobin saturation decreases slightly with decrements in P_{O_2}; loading of oxygen at the alveolar level is therefore affected minimally with mild-to-moderate degrees of hypoxemia. The steeper slope at the lower end of the curve means that, as the hemoglobin becomes desaturated, arterial P_{O_2} drops only minimally, thereby maintaining a gradient favoring oxygen diffusion into tissue cells. Acidosis, a rise in P_{CO_2}, and elevation of temperature all shift the curve to the right, which enhances tissue oxygen uptake. Red blood cell organic phosphates, particularly 2,3 diphosphoglycerate (DPG), also affect the dissociation curve. Banked blood, low in 2,3 DPG, shifts the curve to the left and therefore decreases tissue oxygen uptake. 2,3 DPG levels increase with chronic hypoxia. Chronic lung disease, therefore, results in a shift of the curve to the right, enhancing oxygen delivery to peripheral tissues.

53. The answer is C. *(Schwartz, ed 5. pp 473–475.)* Anticipation and early aggressive treatment of pulmonary insufficiency by mechanical ventilatory support are critical in managing the seriously ill patient. Readily measured changes that can be used to determine either the need for intubation or the appropriate time for weaning from mechanical respiratory support include arterial blood gas levels, dead space/tidal volume ratio (V_D/V_T), alveolar-arterial oxygen tension difference $(A\text{-}a)d_{O_2}$, vital capacity, and respiratory rate. Indications for mechanical ventilation include a respiratory rate over 35/min, vital capacity less than 15 ml/kg, $(A\text{-}a)d_{O_2}$ greater than 350 torr after 15 minutes on 100% oxygen, V_D/V_T greater than 0.6, P_{O_2} less than 60 torr, and a P_{CO_2} greater than 60 torr.

54. The answer is B. *(Hardy, ed 2. pp 252–253.)* Nitrous oxide (N_2O) has a low solubility compared with other inhalation anesthetics. Its blood : gas partition coefficient is 0.47, and it is 30 times more soluble in blood than is nitrogen (N_2). N_2O is also the only anesthetic gas less dense than air. As a result of these properties, nitrous oxide may cause progressive distension of air-filled spaces during prolonged anesthesia. This can lead to undesirable situations whenever there is a pneumothorax, intestinal obstruction, or when procedures like pneumoventriculography (in which the intracranial air space is not free to expand in response to the diffusion of gas into the ventricles) are performed. In each of these cases the N_2O diffuses into the gas-filled compartment faster than N_2 can diffuse out. Since the typical mixture of ingested air (or pneumothorax air) is 80% N_2 and the usual mixture of nitrous oxide anesthetic gas is 80% N_2O, rapid increase in the size of the gas-filled chambers with potentially serious consequences may occur.

55. The answer is C. *(Schwartz, ed 5. pp 160–164.)* In traumatized patients the oxygen dissociation curve is shifted to the left as a result of alkalosis and decreased levels of 2,3 diphosphoglycerate (2,3 DPG) in red blood cells. Correction of the alkalosis and use of frozen erythrocytes that are high in 2,3 DPG (unlike banked blood) will improve release of oxygen by red blood cells to the tissues. While free hemoglobin can be used as an oxygen carrier, coagulopathy results from reduced activity of plasma factors V and VIII. Free myoglobin produces renal tubular damage and does not enhance tissue oxygenation. Although the use of oxygenated fluorocarbons as blood substitutes is under investigation, they are not currently useful clinically because of poor CO_2 diffusion and damage to pulmonary parenchyma.

56. The answer is D. *(Schwartz, ed 5. pp 151–152.)* Adult respiratory distress syndrome (ARDS) has been called "shock lung" or "traumatic wet lung" and occurs under a variety of circumstances. Clinically, its manifestations can range from minimal dysfunction to unrelenting pulmonary failure. Three major physiologic alterations include (1) hypoxemia usually unresponsive to elevations of inspired oxygen concentration; (2) decreased pulmonary compliance, as the lungs become progressively "stiffer" and harder to ventilate; and (3) decreased functional residual capacity. Progressive alveolar collapse occurs owing to leakage of protein-rich fluid into the interstitium and the alveolar spaces with the subsequent radiologic picture of diffuse, fluffy infiltrates bilaterally. Ventilation abnormalities develop that result in shunt formation, decreased resting lung volume, and increased dead space ventilation.

57. The answer is D. *(Schwartz, ed 5. pp 510–518.)* Monitoring of the surgical patient with the Swan-Ganz catheter has become an integral part in the management of operative and postoperative cardiopulmonary hemodynamics in regard to pharmacologic support and fluid balance. Measured parameters such as right and left atrial pressures, right ventricular pressure, pulmonary artery pressure, and capillary wedge pressure, as well as cardiac outputs can all be obtained with right heart catheterization. The catheter can also be used for obtaining mixed venous blood samples, injecting indicator, and infusion of medications. Pulmonary vascular resistance is a calculated value determined from the cardiac output and pressure differential across the right heart. It is not a directly measured value.

58. The answer is A. *(Schwartz, ed 5. pp 463–465.)* The possibility of systemic toxicity is an important concept to remember with the administration of local nerve blocks and results from high blood levels of local anesthetics. The high blood levels may be the result of using total dosages exceeding the recognized safe limits, injection of the local anesthetic into a highly vascular area, or intravenous administration. Local vasodilation occurs in the injected area. Toxic reactions often involve either the cardiovascular system or central nervous system. Severe myocardial depression can occur accompanied by hypotension and bradycardia. Treatment consists of fluid administration and vasopressors. Central nervous system toxicity can be manifested by uncontrolled twitchings or convulsions. Therapy consists of intravenous diazepam (Valium). An acidotic environment, such as the fluid in an abscess cavity, has been shown to render ineffective the anesthetic potential of the various local agents.

59. The answer is C. *(Schwartz, ed 5. pp 165–169.)* A ruptured abdominal aneurysm is a surgical emergency often accompanied by serious hypotension and vascular collapse before surgery and massive fluid shifts with renal failure after surgery. In this case, all the hemodynamic parameters indicate inadequate intravascular volume, and the patient is therefore suffering from hypovolemic hypotension. The low urine output indicates poor renal perfusion, while the high urine specific gravity indicates adequate renal function with compensatory free water conservation. The administration of a vasopressor agent would certainly raise the blood pressure, but it would do so by increasing peripheral vascular resistance, thereby further decreasing tissue perfusion. The deleterious effects of shock would be increased. A vasodilating agent to lower the systemic vascular resistance would lead to profound hypotension and possibly complete vascular collapse because of pooling of an already depleted vascular volume. This patient's blood pressure is critically dependent on an elevated systemic vascular resistance. To properly treat this patient, rapid fluid infusion and expansion of the intravascular volume must be undertaken. This can be easily done with lactated Ringer's solution or blood (or both) until improvements in such parameters as the pulmonary capillary wedge pressure, urine output, and blood pressure are noted.

60. The answer is A. *(Schwartz, ed 5. pp 170–172.)* The patient has now developed clinical evidence of myocardial dysfunction and pump failure. Because of poor myocardial contractility there is a low cardiac output and high pulmonary wedge pressure. Often with myocardial injury there is a difference in the functional reserve of either ventricle. Central venous pressure measurements become unreliable, and now dependence must be placed on pulmonary artery and pulmonary wedge pressures. Since myocardial damage severe enough to cause hypotension has developed, pharmacologic intervention with an inotropic agent is indicated. The use of dopamine may result in an increase in cardiac output with a concomitant improvement in systemic blood pressure, wedge pressure, and urine output. If the patient then stabilizes, consideration can be given to digitalization. The blood pressure is too low to tolerate the use of a vasodilating agent as an afterload reducer at this time. Continued fluid administration would result in further myocardial depression (owing to ventricular overdistension) and the formation of pulmonary edema.

61. The answer is D. *(Miller, ed 2. p 1105. Thoren, Anesth Analg 67:687, 1988.)* Thoracic epidural narcotics have become an increasingly popular means of providing postoperative pain relief in thoracic and upper abdominal surgery. Local action on gamma opiate receptors ensures pain relief and consequent improvement in respiration without vasodilation or paralysis. The less lipid-soluble opiates are effective for long periods. Their slow absorption into the circulation also ensures a low incidence of centrally mediated side effects, such as respiratory depression or generalized itching. When these do occur, the intravenous injection of an opiate antagonist is an effective antidote. The locally mediated analgesia is not affected. One poorly understood side effect, which is apparently unrelated to systemic levels, is a profound reduction in gastric activity. This may be an important consideration after thoracic surgery when an early resumption of oral intake is anticipated.

62–63. The answers are: 62-A (1, 2, 3), 63-B (1, 3). *(Braunwald, ed 11. p 47. Ngai, N Engl J Med 282:541, 1970.)* The cause of malignant hyperthermia is unknown; it may develop in an otherwise healthy young man who has tolerated previous surgery without incident. It should be suspected in the presence of a history of unexplained fever, muscle or connective tissue disorder, or a positive family history (evidence suggests an autosomal dominant inheritance pattern). In addition to fever during anesthesia, the syndrome includes tachycardia, increased O_2 consumption, increased CO_2 production, increased serum K^+, myoglobinuria, and acidosis. Rigidity rather than relaxation following succinylcholine injection may be the first clue to its presence. Investigations have shown excess calcium in myoplasm in patients with the disorder.

If reoperation is necessary, one should premedicate heavily, alkalinize the urine, and avoid depolarizing agents such as succinylcholine. Pretreatment for 24 hours with dantrolene is helpful; it is thought to act directly on muscle fiber to attenuate calcium release.

64. The answer is E (all). *(Schwartz, ed 5. pp 510–515.)* Determination of CVP is an integral part of the overall hemodynamic assessment of the patient. This pressure can be affected by a variety of factors including those of cardiac, noncardiac, and artifactual origin. Venous tone, right ventricular compliance, intrathoracic pressure, and blood volume all influence CVP. Vasoconstrictor drugs, positive pressure ventilation (with and without PEEP), mediastinal compression, and hypervolemia all increase CVP.

65. The answer is D (4). *(Schwartz, ed 5. pp 1573–1575.)* Clinical manifestations of adrenocortical insufficiency include hyperkalemia, hyponatremia, hypoglycemia, fever, weight loss, and dehydration. There is excessive sodium loss in the urine, contraction of the plasma volume, and perhaps hypotension or shock. Classic hyperpigmentation is present in *chronic* Addison's disease only. Addison's disease may present in newborns as a congenital atrophy, as an insidious chronic state often due to tuberculosis, as an acute dysfunction secondary to trauma or adrenal hemorrhage, or as a semiacute adrenal insufficiency seen during stress or surgery. In this last instance, signs and symptoms include nausea, lassitude, vomiting, fever, progressive salt wasting, hyperkalemia, and hypoglycemia. It may be confirmed by measurements of urinary Na^+ loss and absence of response to ACTH.

66. The answer is A (1, 2, 3). *(Hardy, ed 2. pp 147–149.)* Securing a stable airway is one of the most fundamental and important aspects of the management of the severely injured patient. The level of control required will vary from a simple oropharyngeal airway to tracheostomy, depending on the clinical situation. Full control of the airway should be secured in the emergency room if the patient is unstable. Endotracheal intubation will usually be the method chosen, but one should be prepared to do a tracheotomy if attempts at peroral or pernasal intubation are failing or are impractical because of maxillofacial injuries. The most dangerous period is just prior to and during the initial attempts to get control of the airway. Manipulation of the oronasopharynx may provoke combative behavior or vomiting in a patient already confused by drugs, alcohol, hypoxia, or cerebral trauma. The risk of aspiration is high during these initial attempts, and one should make no assumptions about the state of the contents of the patient's stomach. Antacids are recommended just prior to the intubation attempt, if feasible. Although steroids have been recommended in the past, they are no longer considered of value in the management of aspiration of acid gastric juice. The best management requires prevention of the complication of aspiration. In a reasonably cooperative patient awake intubation with topical anesthesia may help to avoid some of the risks of hypotension, arrhythmia, and aspiration associated with the induction of anesthesia. If awake intubation is inappropriate, then an alternative is rapid sequence induction with a thiobarbiturate followed by muscle paralysis with succinylcholine. If elevated intracranial pressure is suspected, or in the presence of a penetrating eye injury, awake intubation is contraindicated.

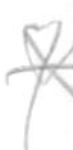

67. The answer is C (2, 4). *(Shoemaker, pp 39–41.)* The metabolic and physiologic effects of drowning and near-drowning depend upon variables that include fluid temperature, extent of aspiration, and whether the aspirate is fresh water or sea water. Cold-water submersion decreases oxygen consumption and results in preferential shunting of blood flow to the heart and brain. This shunting prolongs the period of submersion that can be endured without irreversible cerebral damage. Return of normal cerebral function after as long as 40 minutes of submersion in extremely cold water has been reported. One should also remember that cooling below 30°C will often cause cardiac arrhythmias. Ten percent of affected patients do not aspirate fluid but succumb to asphyxia because of breath holding or laryngospasm. Seventy percent have a significant metabolic acidosis requiring administration of sodium bicarbonate. Significant electrolyte and blood volume changes may or may not be present, depending on the degree of aspiration and toxicity of the fluid medium. Renal damage may occur as a result of hemoglobinuria (from hemolysis), acidosis, hypoxia, or changes in renal blood flow. The most important initial treatment of drowning victims is ventilation. Mouth-to-mouth or mouth-to-nose ventilation should be begun as soon as possible. Corticosteroids and prophylactic antibiotics are not recommended for the prevention of pulmonary complications. However, some workers feel that steroids may be of value in managing the complication of cerebral edema.

68. The answer is A (1, 2, 3). *(Schwartz, ed 5. pp 201–202.)* The most clinically significant clostridial organism is *Clostridium perfringens*. Muscles infected by this organism undergo myonecrosis owing to the action of a necrotizing, hemolytic exotoxin. Treatment consists of rapid incision and drainage of involved areas and penicillin administration in large doses. Good results have been obtained with the use of hyperbaric oxygen as an adjunct to surgical and antimicrobial therapies. Antitoxin is of no benefit either prophylactically or therapeutically.

69. The answer is E (all). *(Braunwald, ed 11. pp 843, 1050, 1491–1492.)* Humans have evolved a highly efficient oxygen transport system that maximizes delivery to peripheral tissues. The acidosis and relative hyperthermia present in peripheral tissues both favor the unloading of hemoglobin-bound oxygen (raise the P_{50}). Conversely, alkalosis and hypothermia result in more avid binding of oxygen by hemoglobin (lower the P_{50}). Alkalosis facilitates oxygen uptake at the lungs but impairs oxygen delivery to tissues. 2,3 Diphosphoglycerate (2,3 DPG) facilitates oxygen release at peripheral tissues. However, transfused blood that has been stored in the traditional anticoagulant, acid citrate dextrose, having been depleted of 2,3 DPG, is relatively ineffective in providing oxygen release. Carbon monoxide preferentially binds to hemoglobin and thus impedes oxygen transport. In addition, it lowers the P_{50} and impairs release of the oxygen that is bound to hemoglobin.

70. The answer is D (4). *(Schwartz, ed 5. p 133.)* The risk of developing viral hepatitis after transfusion is approximately 0.5 percent. The incubation period of hepatitis A is 15 to 50 days and of hepatitis B, 30 to 160 days. While human immune serum globulin prevents type A hepatitis, the results in preventing type B hepatitis are less consistent. Other diseases transmitted by blood transfusion include AIDS, malaria, syphilis, Chagas' disease, and brucellosis. Infusion of human serum albumin probably carries little risk of hepatitis.

71. The answer is E (all). *(Schwartz, ed 5. pp 151–156.)* Abnormalities of ventilation-perfusion ratio result from the shunting of blood to a hypoventilated lung or from the ventilation of hypoperfused regions of lung tissue. Common predisposing factors in the postoperative patient that contribute to this maldistribution include the assumption of a supine position, thoracic and upper abdominal incisions, obesity, atelectasis, and reduced cardiac output.

72. The answer is A (1, 2, 3). *(Schwartz, ed 5. pp 151–156.)* Many factors are responsible for those lung changes leading to pulmonary insufficiency that occur with nonthoracic trauma. Among these factors are microembolization of platelet aggregates, fat particles or debris from infused blood, oxygen toxicity, loss of pulmonary surfactant with subsequent alveolar collapse, sepsis, fluid overload, aspiration, and release of vasoactive substances into the pulmonary circulation. Treatment and prophylaxis include the use of micropore filters, diuretics, positive end-expiratory pressure ventilation (PEEP), holding inspired $F_{I_{O_2}}$ to less than 0.45, treatment of sepsis, and early use of corticosteroids for aspiration and fat embolization.

73. The answer is B (1, 3). *(Shoemaker, pp 319, 370.)* Respiratory benefits of PEEP include an increase in functional residual capacity and decrease in intrapulmonary shunting resulting in improved arterial oxygen tension. PEEP can be increased as long as carefully monitored arterial oxygenation can be shown to increase and as long as cardiovascular depression does not occur. In addition to observation of the blood pressure and arterial oxygen saturation, a pulmonary artery catheter is extremely helpful in measuring directly the effect of the PEEP on the cardiac output.

The mechanism by which PEEP affects the heart is complex. However, a decrease in stroke volume (possibly by decreased left ventricular preload) is thought to be the primary means by which PEEP decreases cardiac output. PEEP also appears to reduce left ventricular compliance, perhaps by its effect on increasing the volume of the surrounding pulmonary tissue.

74. The answer is A (1, 2, 3). *(Zikria, Ann Surg 181:151–156, 1975.)* Smoke inhalation injuries (''smoke poisoning'') and asphyxia account for almost one third of all fire fatalities. As opposed to respiratory burns, which are thermal injuries of the upper respiratory tract, smoke inhalation is a chemical injury to the distal tracheobronchial tree and alveoli. Most patients admitted for this injury have elevated carbon monoxide levels, but a minority will have physical evidence of skin burns (20 percent) or of oropharyngeal burns (25 percent). Visible damage to the respiratory tract is not a frequent finding. Chest films initially are often negative even in those patients who subsequently develop respiratory failure from pulmonary edema or pneumonitis. Patients with elevated carboxyhemoglobin levels or evidence of smoke inhalation should be hospitalized for a minimum of 24 hr for observation regardless of normal arterial blood gases and chest x-ray.

75. The answer is B (1, 3). *(Sabiston, ed 13. p 1332.)* Gastric aspiration is best treated by tracheal suctioning, oxygen, and positive pressure ventilation. Bronchoscopy is helpful if particulate matter is causing bronchial obstruction or if the vomitus is found to contain particulate material. Bronchial lavage is no longer recommended, and steroids and prophylactic antibiotics have not been shown to be of value.

76. The answer is A (1, 2, 3). *(Sabiston, ed 13. pp 2001–2002.)* Although tracheostomy is occasionally an emergency procedure, it can be more effectively performed in an operating room where hemostasis and antisepsis are readily achieved. Most authorities recommend a horizontal incision; however, limited direct midline incisions have the advantage of not opening any unnecessary tissue planes and perhaps reducing the incidence of bleeding complications. Both approaches have advocates. In either case, the incision is made just below the cricoid cartilage, the strap muscles are spared and retracted, the thyroid isthmus is divided, if necessary, and the trachea is entered at the second tracheal ring. The second and third tracheal rings are incised vertically, allowing placement of the tracheostomy tube. The first tracheal ring and the cricoid cartilage must be left intact.

77. The answer is C (2, 4). *(Sabiston, ed 13. p 95.)* For all surgical patients the risk of a postoperative myocardial infarction is about 0.15 percent. However, the incidence has been reported as high as ten times that for patients over 70 years of age. One third of patients undergoing general anesthesia and being operated on within 3 months of a previous myocardial infarction suffers another infarction. If surgery is delayed until 6 months after the initial infarction, then the subsequent rate of reinfarction approaches only 4 to 5 percent. Stable angina and moderate degrees of hypertension have not been found to be associated with higher rates of infarction.

78–80. The answers are: 78-A, 79-B, 80-B. *(Hardy, ed 2. pp 250–255.)* Curare and pancuronium are nondepolarizing agents that bind competitively. Myasthenics are very sensitive to curare. Succinylcholine is attractive because of its rapid (depolarizing) action, but it may cause transient hyperkalemia: since succinylcholine causes depolarization of skeletal muscles, potassium is released from the muscle into the circulation. In patients with massive crush injuries or burns in which cellular release of potassium may already be high, the administration of succinylcholine will further exacerbate the hyperkalemia and lead to ventricular fibrillation. One in 3000 patients suffers prolonged action of succinylcholine because of an abnormally weak cholinesterase activity.

81–85. The answers are: 81-C, 82-A, 83-B, 84-C, 85-D. *(Schwartz, ed 5. pp 174–176.)* The initial profile of gram negative sepsis is dependent on the patient's volume status. The normovolemic patient will enter a hyperdynamic state characterized by a high cardiac output with a decreased peripheral vascular resistance, while the hypovolemic patient will maintain a low cardiac output with increased peripheral vascular resistance. Hypotension is present in both situations as is an early respiratory alkalosis secondary to hyperventilation, which is replaced by a metabolic acidosis if the septic state goes untreated. Treatment centers around resolving the sepsis either with antibiotics or antibiotics in conjunction with surgical drainage. Aggressive fluid replacement and pulmonary support are also extremely important. The use of vasopressors should not be used in place of aggressive volume replacement because this will elevate the blood pressure but at the expense of perfusion to vital organs.

86–89. The answers are: 86-C, 87-D, 88-E, 89-A. *(Hardy, ed 2. pp 250–255.)* Nitrous oxide (N_2O) is a frequently used inhalation analgesic. However, because the MAC (minimum alveolar anesthetic concentration) is so high (over 100), true anesthesia at one atmosphere pressure cannot be obtained without compromising oxygen delivery to the patient. Since nitrous oxide is thirty times more soluble than nitrogen in blood, it enters a collection of trapped air at a rate faster than nitrogen leaves the collection. Thus, the trapped air will increase in volume. If the trapped air is a result of bowel obstruction, intestinal distension will increase.

Halothane is a very potent inhalation anesthetic with an MAC of 0.75. Cardiovascular depression results from a number of different mechanisms. Hypotension and decreased cardiac output have been associated with a direct depression of myocardial muscle fibers and peripheral vascular smooth muscle fibers. An effect on the medullary vasomotor centers as well as on sympathetic ganglionic transmissions to the heart has been reported.

Enflurane is a halogenated inhalation anesthetic with an MAC of 1.2. It is similar to halothane in its anesthetic characteristics. However, in a small number of normal patients it may induce electroencephalographic changes similar to those seen in epilepsy.

Methoxyflurane is the most potent and least volatile halogenated inhalation anesthetic with an MAC of 0.16. Its clinical use has been curtailed because of the high risk of nephrotoxicity of the free fluoride ions released during its biodegradation.

Morphine is a potent narcotic agent. Its use during general anesthesia can potentiate the analgesic effects of the inhalation agents. It causes histamine release with the risk of hypotension if given in a large bolus dose.

90–93. The answers are: 90-D, 91-C, 92-B, 93-A. *(Schwartz, ed 5. pp 120–121.)* Prothrombin time measures the speed of coagulation in the extrinsic pathway. A tissue source of procoagulant (thromboplastin) with calcium is added to plasma. The test will detect deficiencies in factors II, V, VII, X, and fibrinogen and is used to monitor patients receiving coumarin derivatives. However, even small amounts of heparin will artificially prolong the clotting time so that accurate prothrombin times can only be obtained when the patient has not received heparin for at least 5 hours.

The intrinsic pathway is measured by the partial thromboplastin time. This test is sensitive for defects in factors VIII, IX, XI, XII, and all the factors of the extrinsic pathway and is used to monitor the status of patients on heparin.

The bleeding time assesses the interaction of platelets and the formation of the platelet plug. Therefore it will pick up deficiencies in both qualitative and quantitative platelet function. Ingestion of aspirin within 1 week of the test will alter the result.

The thrombin time assesses qualitative abnormalities in fibrinogen and the presence of inhibitors to fibrin polymerization. A standard amount of fibrin is added to a fixed volume of plasma and clotting time is measured.

Skin: Wounds, Infections, Burns; Hands; and Plastic Surgery

DIRECTIONS: Each question below contains five suggested responses. Select the **one best** response to each question.

94. Split thickness skin grafts differ from full thickness grafts in that the split thickness grafts

(A) contain no dermal elements
(B) provide more flexibility and strength
(C) develop deeper pigmentation following transfer
(D) are more cosmetically acceptable
(E) fail more readily if a recipient's bed conditions are suboptimal

95. A 20-year-old man sustains a deep laceration on the volar surface of the right wrist. Median nerve injury would result in

(A) a claw hand defect
(B) a wrist drop
(C) a sensory deficit only
(D) an inability to oppose the thumb to the other fingers
(E) an inability to flex the metacarpophalangeal joints

96. All the following statements are true EXCEPT

(A) a dehisced wound that is resutured gains strength faster than a primary wound
(B) wounds heal faster at 39°C (102.2°F) than at 37°C (98.6°F)
(C) wound healing is accelerated in an environment of low tissue oxygen
(D) synthesis of new collagen is blocked during periods of deficiency of ascorbic acid
(E) wound healing will not occur normally in the absence of monocytes

97. Although wide surgical excision is the traditional treatment for malignant melanoma, narrow excision of thin (less than 1 mm deep) stage I melanomas has been found to be equally safe and effective when the margin of resection is as small as

(A) 3 mm
(B) 5 mm
(C) 1 cm
(D) 3 cm
(E) 5 cm

---

98. A 50-year-old man presented with a single firm, nontender, movable subcutaneous mass in his right side. The lesion, shown below, was excised. Microscopic examination disclosed a tumor containing palisade spindle cells, Verocay bodies, and a peripheral nerve at one edge. The next step in the management of this patient is to

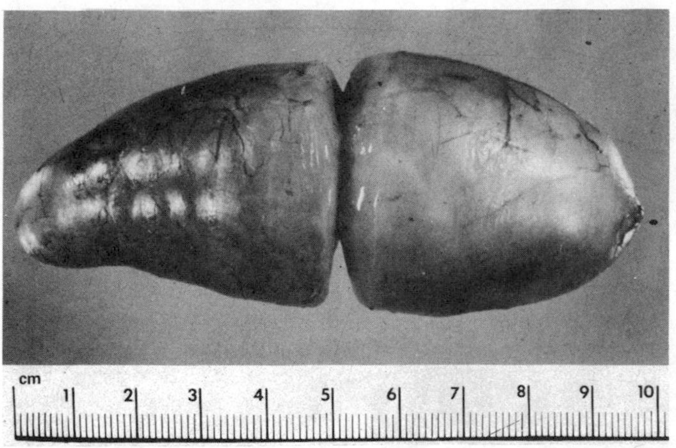

(A) reexcise the area for wider margins
(B) order a myelogram for nerve root evaluation
(C) reexamine him for café au lait spots
(D) counsel him on the genetic implications of the lesion
(E) assure him that the surgery was curative

99. Proper treatment for frostbite consists of

(A) debridement of the affected part followed by silver sulfadiazine dressings
(B) administration of corticosteroids
(C) administration of vasodilators
(D) immersion of the affected part in water at 40°C to 44°C (104°F to 111.2°F)
(E) rewarming of the affected part at room temperature

---

100. A 65-year-old woman presents with the massive scalp tumor shown below, which has been present for over 25 years. The most likely route of spread of this tumor is

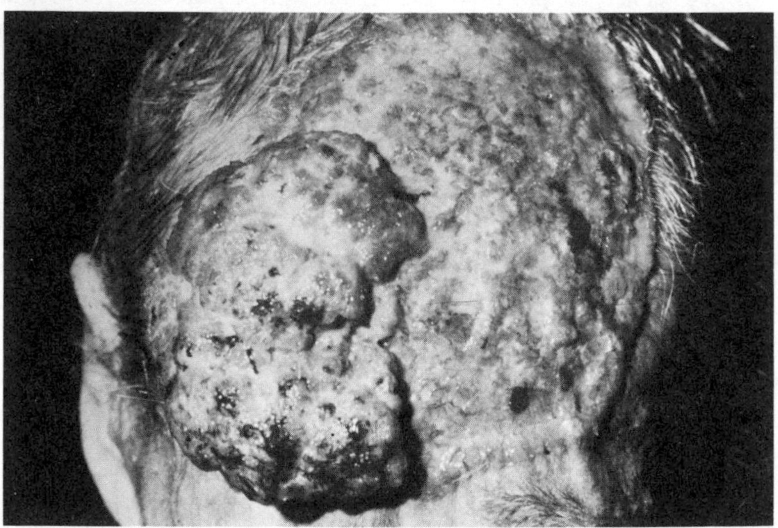

(A) blood-borne metastasis
(B) lymph node metastasis
(C) perineural invasion
(D) local invasion
(E) none of the above

DIRECTIONS: Each question below contains four suggested responses of which **one or more** is correct. Select

A	if	**1, 2, and 3**	are correct
B	if	**1 and 3**	are correct
C	if	**2 and 4**	are correct
D	if	**4**	is correct
E	if	**1, 2, 3, and 4**	are correct

101. Although the likelihood of a nevus' becoming malignant is difficult to predict accurately, excisional biopsy is recommended for the management of

(1) congenital nevus
(2) junctional nevus
(3) juvenile nevus
(4) intradermal nevus

102. Correct statements regarding the carpal tunnel syndrome include which of the following?

(1) It is often secondary to a wrist fracture
(2) It may be associated with pregnancy
(3) It may cause nocturnal dysesthesia
(4) It is often associated with vascular compromise

103. A 60-year-old woman presents with the skin lesion shown below, which had been present for 10 years. She reported a history of radiation treatments to that hand for "eczema." Correct statements concerning this lesion include

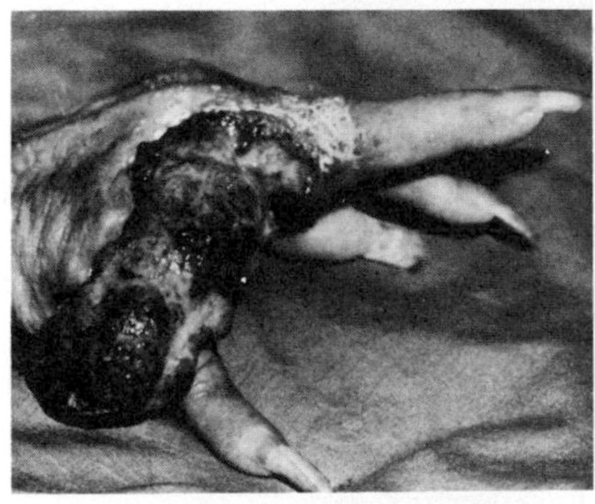

(1) it is more malignant than basal cell carcinoma
(2) it occurs more frequently in blondes
(3) it often metastasizes to regional lymph nodes
(4) it should be treated by radiation therapy

SUMMARY OF DIRECTIONS

A	B	C	D	E
1,2,3 only	1,3 only	2,4 only	4 only	All are correct

104. Toxic shock syndrome, believed to be caused by staphylococcal endotoxemia, comprises a constellation of symptoms and signs that must include

(1) rash
(2) fever
(3) desquamation
(4) hypotension

105. An 8-lb infant, born following uncomplicated labor and delivery, is noted to have a unilateral cleft lip and palate. The parents should be advised that

(1) the child almost certainly has other congenital anomalies
(2) rehabilitation requires adjunctive speech and hearing therapy
(3) lip repair is indicated at 1 year of age
(4) palate repair is indicated between 1 and 1½ years of age

106. Management of leukoplakia of the oral cavity includes

(1) excisional biopsy of all lesions
(2) improvement of oral hygiene
(3) low-dose radiation therapy
(4) ascertaining that dentures fit properly

107. True statements about thyroglossal duct sinus or cyst include which of the following?

(1) It may become infected and require drainage
(2) It may undergo malignant change
(3) It is more likely to recur if the central hyoid segment is not removed
(4) It usually becomes clinically significant in childhood

108. Correct statements regarding laryngeal cancer include which of the following?

(1) There is a statistically significant association with smoking
(2) Stage 1 lesions of the true vocal cords have a 50 percent 5-year survival
(3) A high percentage of affected patients are alcoholic
(4) Laryngectomy is an essential part of management for stage 1 and stage 2 lesions

109. A 40-year-old woman undergoes wide excision of a pigmented lesion of her thigh. Pathologic examination reveals malignant melanoma that is Clark's level IV. Examination of the groin is normal. The patient should be advised that

(1) radiotherapy will be an important part of subsequent therapy
(2) the likelihood of groin node metastases is remote
(3) immunotherapy is an effective form of adjunctive treatment for metastatic malignant melanoma
(4) groin dissection is not indicated unless and until groin nodes become palpable

110. A 30-year-old man is struck in the right periorbital area by an assailant. On his arrival in the emergency room, he displays findings compatible with a blow-out fracture of the orbit. Such findings would include which of the following?

(1) Vertical gaze diplopia
(2) Right nasolabial anesthesia
(3) Enophthalmos
(4) Paralysis of upward gaze on the right side

111. Correct statements concerning injuries to the hand include which of the following?

(1) Extensor tendon injuries have a better prognosis than flexor tendon injuries
(2) Mallet finger is caused by fracture of a distal phalanx at the point of extensor tendon insertion
(3) Boutonniere (buttonhole) deformity is caused by injury to the extensor tendon near its insertion into the middle phalanx
(4) Zone I (distal finger) tendon repairs are associated with a better prognosis than zone II (''no-man's land'') tendon repair

112. True statements regarding perichondritis of the pinna include which of the following?

(1) It can be complicated by extensive loss of cartilage
(2) Wound culture and sensitivity testing is mandatory
(3) Wide incision and drainage is indicated
(4) Antibiotics are indicated

DIRECTIONS: Each group of questions below consists of four lettered headings followed by a set of numbered items. For each numbered item select

A	if the item is associated with	(A) **only**
B	if the item is associated with	(B) **only**
C	if the item is associated with	**both** (A) and (B)
D	if the item is associated with	**neither** (A) nor (B)

Each lettered heading may be used **once, more than once, or not at all.**

Questions 113–115

(A) Basal cell carcinoma
(B) Squamous cell carcinoma
(C) Both
(D) Neither

113. Predominant occurrence in exposed areas, most frequently in weather-beaten skin

114. Improved survival when excision is accompanied by prophylactic lymph node dissection

115. Rare metastasis, even when primary lesion is locally advanced

Questions 116–118

(A) Clostridial cellulitis
(B) Clostridial myonecrosis
(C) Both
(D) Neither

116. Crepitus

117. Usually mild systemic effects

118. Characterized by rapid invasion of uninjured tissue

Skin: Wounds, Infections, Burns; Hands; and Plastic Surgery

Answers

94. The answer is C. *(Davis, pp 3138–3142.)* Free grafts are defined as full thickness if the entire thickness of skin, including both epidermis and dermis, is transferred, and as split thickness if the epidermis and only a portion of dermis are transferred. Some nutrient diffusion is essential to graft survival. It is clear that the thinner the graft, the better the take, particularly in the presence of mechanical barriers, such as infected tissue and blood, that produce a suboptimal recipient bed. Strength, flexibility, and appearance are qualities provided by the dermis. When cosmetic considerations become important, as in facial wounds, full thickness grafts are necessary to provide satisfactory skin color, texture, and thickness. Split thickness skin grafts are more likely to develop deep pigmentation during the first 6 to 9 months following transfer; patients receiving the split thickness grafts should be advised to avoid solar radiation during this period.

95. The answer is D. *(Davis, pp 2350–2351.)* Median nerve injury at the wrist level results in paralysis of the thenar muscles that position the thumb for opposition to the other fingers. A claw hand and paralysis of intrinsic flexor hand muscles indicate a problem associated with ulnar nerve injury; a wrist drop results from radial nerve injury.

96. The answer is C. *(Davis, pp 461–504.)* Wound healing is decreased, both in rate and in tensile strength, by a decrease in oxygen tension. Therefore, it is important for the patient to have good oxygenation and an adequate hemoglobin. When a normally healing wound is disrupted and resutured, the return of tensile strength is so rapid that the burst strength is nearly what it would have been had the dehiscence not occurred. Wounds heal faster at higher temperatures because of increased blood flow and metabolic rate. Scars appear to undergo remodeling as long as 30 years after injury. There exists an equilibrium between collagen synthesis and collagen destruction that results in this remodeling process. Vitamin C deficiency blocks the synthesis of new collagen, thus destroying the equilibrium and causing disruption of wounds that had healed perfectly months before. Inflammation is necessary for wound healing. The release of various amines from mast cells, the perfusion of capillaries, and accumulation of white cells, especially monocytes and macrophages, are important in providing the best milieu for repair to proceed.

97. The answer is C. *(Veronesi, N Engl J Med 318:1159–1162, 1988.)* Wide excision of melanomas, with margins of 3 to 5 cm beyond the lateral edges of tumor, has traditionally been considered mandatory. A 5-year prospective multicenter study involving over 600 randomly assigned patients with thin stage I melanomas, however, showed that local recurrence rates, as well as the subsequent development of metastatic disease, was not different when margins of 1 cm or 3 cm were taken, provided that tumor thickness did not exceed 1 mm.

98. The answer is E. *(Davis, pp 1074–1075.)* Solitary schwannomas (neurilemmomas) are benign tumors of nerve sheaths that are asymptomatic unless large enough or so positioned as to compress the involved nerve. These tumors are most often solitary; local excision is usually adequate therapy. Although spinal nerve roots are often involved, there is no reason to evaluate them in the absence of root symptoms. Histologically, schwannomas are composed of spindle cells arranged in interlacing bundles. Sometimes the cells palisade at either end of the bundle of parallel fibers, forming a pattern known as Verocay bodies. In contrast to the neurofibromas of von Recklinghausen's disease, solitary schwannomas are not associated with skin pigment changes (café au lait spots) or with any recognized inheritance pattern.

99. The answer is D. *(Davis, pp 2929–2933.)* Many methods of treating frostbite have been tried throughout the years. These include massage, warm water immersion, or covering the affected area. Rapid warming by immersion in water slightly above normal body temperature (40–44°C) is the most effective method, however. Because the frostbitten region is numb and especially vulnerable, it should be protected from trauma or excessive heat during treatment. Further treatment may include elevation to minimize edema, administration of antibiotics and tetanus toxoid, and debridement of necrotic skin as needed.

100. The answer is D. *(Davis, p 2410. Schwartz, ed 5. p 538.)* The patient has a basal cell carcinoma, which is a tumor that rarely metastasizes. These tumors grow indolently except in immunosuppressed patients or where the tumor extends into a mucous membrane—then rapid extension is the rule and growth becomes truly invasive and malignant. Neglected lesions slowly erode into deep local structures, in this case the skull, orbit, or brain.

101. The answer is B (1, 3). *(Davis, pp 2377–2393.)* Congenital nevi are so designated because they contain pigment at birth. While relatively rare, these lesions have a higher incidence of melanoma than do acquired nevi, which do not form pigment until later in life. The risk of melanoma's developing in a congenital nevus appears to increase with age and the size of the lesion. Congenital nevi should be removed as prophylaxis against melanoma. Juvenile nevi, or ''benign juvenile melanomas,'' are lesions of childhood that bear a close histopathological resemblance to melanoma. Removal for diagnosis is indicated. Acquired nevi are thought to have a very low malignant potential. Acquired nevi are classified according to their location in the dermis. Most nevi of childhood arise at the epidermal-dermal junction (junctional nevi) and appear to grow vertically into the dermis (intradermal nevi) as adulthood approaches.

102. The answer is A (1, 2, 3). *(Davis, pp 2348–2349.)* Signs and symptoms of the carpal tunnel syndrome are related to the distribution of the median nerve. This nerve, which passes through the carpal tunnel in the wrist with the finger flexor tendons, may suffer compression from fibrous scarring or malalignment following a fracture of the wrist. Nerve compression may also occur in patients with rheumatoid arthritis who develop flexor tenosynovitis. In women, the syndrome frequently first appears during pregnancy and recurs during the premenstrual phase of subsequent menstrual cycles. In these cases, symptoms are presumably the result of the effects of fluid retention and pressure on the median nerve owing to tissue swelling. In many instances, symptoms are limited to nocturnal pain and paresthesias.

103. The answer is A (1, 2, 3). *(Schwartz, ed 5. pp 539–540.)* Squamous cell carcinoma occurs in people who have had chronic sun exposure, chronic ulcers or sinus tracts (draining osteomyelitis), and a history of radiation or thermal injury (Margolin's ulcer). It is more malignant than basal cell carcinoma, grows more rapidly, and metastasizes. The lesions occur more frequently in blondes. A radiation-induced carcinoma, or one arising in a burn scar, should not be treated with radiation therapy for fear of further damage.

104. The answer is E (all). *(Landercasper, MMWR 29:441, 1980. Landercasper, Surgery 102:96–98, 1987.)* To meet the Centers for Disease Control case definition of toxic shock syndrome, a patient must exhibit diffuse macular erythroderma; a fever greater than or equal to 102°F; desquamation, particularly of palms and soles; hypotension; and severe derangement of three or more organ systems. Although the initial description of toxic shock syndrome involved patients using menstrual tampons, its occurrence following clean surgical procedures, including breast aspiration and biopsy, is now reported.

105. The answer is C (2, 4). *(Davis, pp 3160–3162.)* Clefts of the lip and palate occur relatively frequently (1 in 750 live births); they may be unilateral or bilateral and can vary from a small notch to a complete cleft of the lip and palate. Most clefts occur as isolated anomalies but occasionally are associated with neurologic, orthopedic, or cardiac anomalies. A frequently recommended protocol for management is lip repair in the first 3 months of life and palate repair at 12 to 18 months. 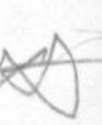
Other cosmetic procedures can be performed late in childhood and adolescence.

Palate repair after 2 years of age is associated with a high incidence of speech impairment; repair in the early months of life can lead to a hazardous loss of blood that is poorly tolerated by the infant. Repair of the lip usually should be accomplished as soon as the infant is sufficiently stabilized to tolerate anesthesia with reasonable safety. Ten to twelve weeks are often recommended as the time for lip repair. At this age, the affected baby usually can be converted to dropper or cup feedings in the postoperative period, thereby facilitating healing of the lip by reducing the need for suckling with the freshly wounded tissues.

106. The answer is C (2, 4). *(Davis, pp 2458–2459.)* White patches in the oral cavity (leukoplakia) sometimes are incorrectly interpreted as a premalignant condition. Microscopic examination of leukoplakia may in fact reveal hyperplasia, keratosis, or dyskeratosis, of which the last finding is the most serious because of its association with malignancy. Only about 5 percent of patients with leukoplakia develop cancer. A suggested treatment protocol for patients with thin lesions advocates a program of strict oral hygiene and avoidance of alcohol and tobacco. Biopsy is reserved only for those with thick lesions (since carcinoma in situ may be present). Radiation therapy is contraindicated. Approximately 50 percent of all oral cancers occur in patients who have associated areas of hyperkeratosis and dyskeratosis.

107. The answer is E (all). *(Davis, pp 1112–1115.)* The embryonic thyroid gland arises at the base of the tongue (foramen cecum) and migrates into the neck. The connection between the cervical thyroid and foramen cecum is usually obliterated. It may persist as a sinus, which assumes clinical importance if it becomes cystic or infected. Clinical identification is usually made in childhood but may first be made in older adults. Complete removal of a thyroglossal duct cyst requires excision of the central portion of the hyoid bone along with the entire thyroglossal duct up to the foramen cecum. If the cyst is large, thyroid scanning should be performed to confirm the presence of functioning thyroid tissue in the usual cervical location. An occasional affected patient will have functioning thyroid tissue only in association with the thyroglossal cyst at the base of the tongue. Papillary carcinomas have occasionally been identified in thyroglossal duct remnants.

108. The answer is B (1, 3). *(Davis, pp 1143–1149.)* Cancer of the larynx occurs in a male-to-female ratio of 11:1 and a definite correlation with smoking has been demonstrated. Alcohol has been implicated as a carcinogen, since up to 40 percent of patients with laryngeal cancer are heavy drinkers. About 56 percent of these epidermoid cancers occur in the glottic region (the area of the true vocal cords) and 42 percent occur in the supraglottic area. Carcinoma of the true cords is easily detected inasmuch as it causes hoarseness. Early therapy should be possible with a 90 percent or better 5-year survival rate. When the cancer is confined to the true cords, radiotherapy is an effective treatment modality. For stage 2, 3, or 4 lesions, laryngectomy is necessary. It is usually performed along with a radical neck dissection on the side of the lesion (even if no nodes are palpable). Using this approach, survivals of about 70 percent have been reported for stage 2 and 3 lesions. Rehabilitation of the patient after laryngectomy is a major problem. Some degree of esophageal speech can be learned by about 75 percent of patients, but only about half of all laryngectomy patients will be able to communicate effectively with strangers and new acquaintances.

109. The answer is D (4). *(Freinkel, JAMA 251:1864–1866, 1984. Schwartz, ed 5. pp 542–546.)* The survival of patients with malignant melanoma correlates with the depth of invasion (Clark) and the thickness of the lesion (Breslow). It is widely held that patients with thin lesions (<0.76 mm) and Clark's level I and II lesions are adequately managed by wide local excision. The incidence of nodal metastases rises with increasing Clark's level of invasion such that a level IV lesion has a 30 to 50 percent incidence of nodal metastases. The assumption that removal of microscopic foci of disease is beneficial, in conjunction with retrospective data indicating improved survival in patients who have undergone removal of clinically negative but pathologically positive nodes, has led to the widely held belief that prophylactic node dissections are indicated for melanoma. Prospective data have challenged this concept. Veronesi and Sim have found that patients undergoing prophylactic node dissections survived no longer than those who were followed closely and underwent node dissections only after nodes became palpable. The subject remains controversial and further study and follow-up are necessary. Immunotherapy has not been successful in controlling widespread metastatic melanoma even when added to chemotherapy. Intralesional administration of BCG has been demonstrated to control local skin lesions in only 20 percent of patients. Dinitrochlorobenzene (DNCB) can also be used.

110. The answer is E (all). *(Davis, pp 1097–1099.)* Fractures of the orbital floor (blow-out fractures) may follow direct trauma to the face. Herniation of the orbital contents into the maxillary antrum causes enophthalmos. Entrapment of the inferior rectus and inferior oblique muscles results in upward gaze diplopia and paralysis of upward gaze. Nasolabial anesthesia results from injury to the infraorbital branch of the trigeminal nerve. Treatment may require open reduction and repair of the orbital floor.

111. The answer is E (all). *(Davis, pp 2305–2308.)* Flexor tendons pass through a fascial tunnel that prevents bowing of the tendon during flexion. Extensor tendons are located in loose areolar tissue. During the healing process, injured or repaired flexor tendons become adherent to nonyielding adjacent fascial structures, thus limiting function. Zone I injuries have a good prognosis because they are located distal to the fascial tunnel. A baseball or football striking the tip of a finger may cause avulsion of the extensor mechanism from its insertion into the distal phalanx, giving rise to a mallet deformity of the finger. It is a challenging injury frequently associated with avulsion fractures of the distal phalanx. Mallet finger often requires internal fixation and carefully directed physiotherapy to prevent long-term disability. Transection of the central extensor tendon near its insertion into the middle phalanx may result in a buttonhole type of defect (boutonniere deformity) through which the proximal interphalangeal (PIP) joint may protrude. The PIP joint takes on an attitude of flexion that may increase when efforts to extend the joint actively are made. The vectors transmitted to the distal interphalangeal joint by the displaced tendons cause a hyperextension of that joint. Repair (if a laceration) and 6 weeks of careful immobilization are important if normal function is to be recovered.

112. The answer is E (all). *(Howard, ed 2. pp 458–459.)* Avascular and septic necrosis of the cartilage of the pinna of the ear results from a collection of pus between the perichondrium and cartilage. The infection tends to be persistent and should be treated by wide incision and drainage together with pressure dressings. The incision should be made just anterior to the antihelix on the lateral surface so that the scar will be minimally conspicuous. Incisions for superficial infections should be avoided, however, because of the danger of inducing perichondritis. Since gram-negative rods are often involved, cultures and sensitivity tests can be very useful. Treatment with systemic antibiotics is indicated in perichondritis.

113–115. The answers are: 113-C, 114-D, 115-A. *(Davis, pp 2408–2418.)* Basal and squamous cell carcinomas are the two most common cancers in humans. Both occur predominantly in areas of chronic inflammation or trauma. Consequently, weather-beaten, irradiated, burned, or tobacco-irritated areas of the head, neck, lips, limbs, and hands are sites of most frequent occurrence. Squamous cell cancers with high-risk features (larger than 2 cm in diameter, poorly differentiated, or present in unhealing wounds such as burn scars) have a 21 to 35 percent incidence of lymph node metastasis when first seen. Otherwise, nodal involvement is unusual and lymph node dissection should be reserved for palpable nodes. Basal cell cancers, by contrast, are extremely low-grade malignancies that rarely metastasize.

116–118. The answers are: 116-C, 117-A, 118-B. *(Schwartz, ed 5. pp 201–202.)* Clostridial cellulitis results from infection of devitalized tissue by predominantly nontoxigenic clostridia species. Subcutaneous gas may be present and spread dramatically along fascial planes; however, uninjured tissue is not invaded, and toxemia is not characteristic of this type of wound infection. Treatment is open drainage, debridement, and anticlostridial antibiotics.

Clostridial myonecrosis, or "gas gangrene," is a life-threatening, invasive infection, usually caused by *C. perfringens* and additional synergistic aerobic and anaerobic bacteria. Crepitus and severe toxemia are common. Extensively contaminated traumatic injuries, including neglected skin lesions in diabetic extremities, are frequent sites of involvement. When no portal of entry can be found, gastrointestinal (especially colonic) neoplasms have been implicated. Treatment consists of aggressive debridement or amputation, high-dose anticlostridial antibiotics, and hyperbaric oxygen in selected cases.

Trauma and Shock

DIRECTIONS: Each question below contains five suggested responses. Select the **one best** response to each question.

119. A 4-year-old child is noted to have fractures of the 10th and 11th ribs on the left side with a falling hematocrit following an automobile accident. Because of evidence of continuing bleeding the patient is taken to the operating room where abdominal exploration discloses a laceration of the lower pole of the spleen. The surgeon should

(A) ligate the splenic artery but leave the spleen in place
(B) perform splenectomy
(C) perform a partial splenectomy
(D) perform a splenorrhaphy (repair of the laceration)
(E) cauterize the spleen and place a drain in the area

120. A 65-year-old man who smokes cigarettes and has chronic obstructive pulmonary disease falls and fractures the 7th, 8th, and 9th ribs in the left anterolateral chest. Chest x-ray is otherwise normal. Appropriate treatment might include all the following EXCEPT

(A) strapping the chest with adhesive tape
(B) postural drainage physiotherapy
(C) intercostal nerve block
(D) abdominal paracentesis
(E) hospitalization

121. Following traumatic peripheral nerve transection, regrowth usually occurs at which of the following rates?

(A) 0.1 mm per day
(B) 1 mm per day
(C) 5 mm per day
(D) 1 cm per day
(E) None of the above

122. A 20-year-old female college student is admitted to a hospital with crampy abdominal pain and vomiting. History reveals that 4 years previously she was in an automobile accident in which she was apparently saved from serious injury by her seat belt. She was discharged from the hospital 4 days after that injury and has had no symptoms until now. Chest x-rays are now obtained and appear below in Figures 1 and 2. After passage of a nasogastric tube, the patient has substantial relief of symptoms. Several days later, she is asymptomatic, and an upper GI series is performed. Figure 3 below shows a selected film from the small bowel follow-through series. The best management at this time is

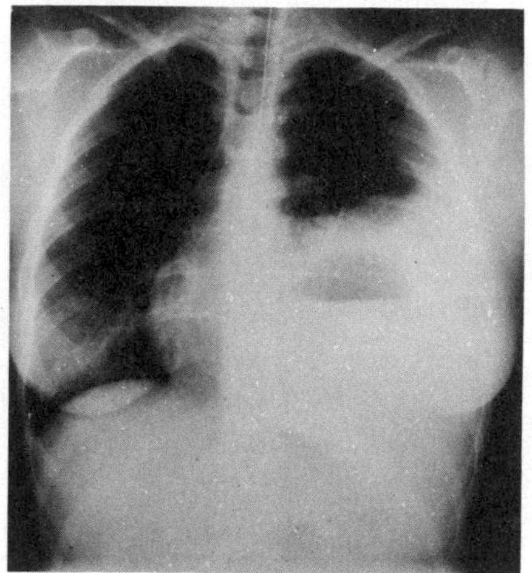

Figure 1

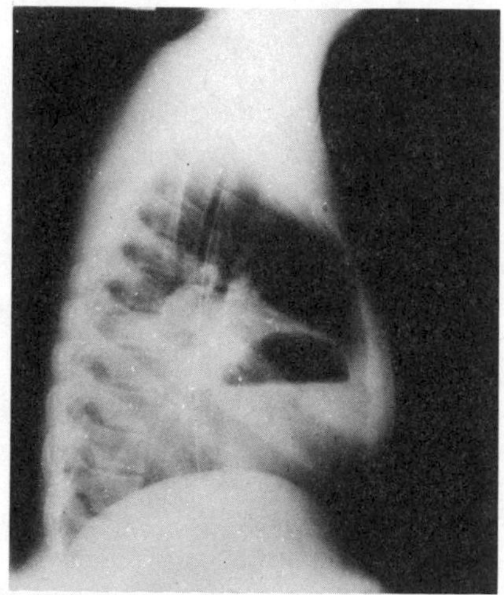

Figure 2

(A) exploration of the patient's abdomen
(B) exploration of the patient's left chest through a thoracotomy incision
(C) a left thoracoabdominal incision preparatory to replacing the diaphragm with a prosthesis
(D) observation, with operation only if symptoms recur and become unmanageable
(E) discharge from the hospital, because recurrence of symptoms is rare and easily treated

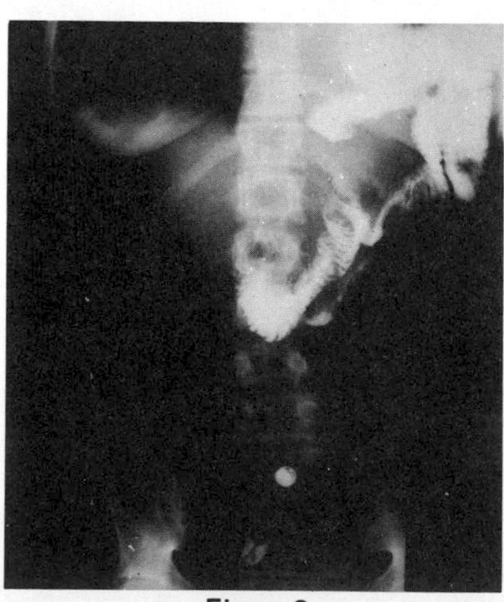

Figure 3

Questions 123–126

A 28-year-old man is brought to the emergency room for a severe head injury after a fall. Initially lethargic, he becomes comatose and does not move his right side. His left pupil is dilated and responds only sluggishly.

123. The most common initial manifestation of increasing intracranial pressure in the victim of head trauma is

(A) change in level of consciousness
(B) ipsilateral (side of hemorrhage) pupillary dilatation
(C) contralateral pupillary dilatation
(D) hemiparesis
(E) hypertension

124. Initial emergency reduction of intracranial pressure is most rapidly accomplished by

(A) saline-furosemide (Lasix) infusion
(B) urea infusion
(C) mannitol infusion
(D) intravenous dexamethasone (Decadron)
(E) hyperventilation

125. This patient's pupillary dilatation is most likely to be the result of compression of which of the following cranial nerves?

(A) Optic
(B) Oculomotor
(C) Trochlear
(D) Ophthalmic branch of the trigeminal
(E) Abducent

126. In the patient described, compression of the affected nerve is produced by

(A) infection within the cavernous sinus
(B) herniation of the uncal process of the temporal lobe
(C) laceration of the corpus callosum by the falx cerebri
(D) occult damage to the superior cervical ganglion
(E) cerebellar hypoxia

127. A 31-year-old man is brought to the emergency room following an automobile accident in which his chest struck the steering wheel. Examination reveals stable vital signs but the patient exhibits multiple palpable rib fractures and paradoxical movement of the right side of the chest. Chest x-ray shows no evidence of pneumothorax or hemothorax, but a large pulmonary contusion is developing. Proper treatment would consist of which of the following?

(A) Tracheostomy, mechanical ventilation, and positive end-expiratory pressure
(B) Stabilization of the chest wall with sandbags
(C) Stabilization with towel clips
(D) Immediate operative stabilization
(E) No treatment unless signs of respiratory distress develop

128. Pulmonary contusion injuries are characterized by all the following EXCEPT

(A) onset within minutes of the injury
(B) resolution within 2 to 5 days
(C) localized area of involvement on chest x-ray
(D) need for substantial volume replacement
(E) need for mechanical ventilatory assistance

129. A 23-year-old, previously healthy man presents to the emergency room after sustaining a single gunshot wound to the left chest. The entrance wound is 3 cm inferior to the nipple and the exit wound just below the scapula. A chest tube is placed and drains 400 ml of blood and continues to drain 50 to 75 ml/hr during the initial resuscitation. Initial blood pressure of 70/0 responds to 2 L crystalloid and is now 100/70. Abdominal examination is unremarkable. Chest x-ray reveals a reexpanded lung and no free air under the diaphragm. The next management step should be

(A) admission and observation
(B) peritoneal lavage
(C) exploratory thoracotomy
(D) exploratory celiotomy
(E) local wound exploration

130. A patient who sustains acute lower cervical transection secondary to cervical fracture dislocation may be expected to demonstrate which of the following manifestations during the early treatment period?

(A) Respiratory failure
(B) Hypertension
(C) Tachycardia
(D) Hypothermia
(E) Hyperreflexia

131. True statements concerning penetrating pancreatic trauma include all the following EXCEPT

(A) the major cause of death is exsanguination from associated vascular injuries
(B) management of a ductal injury to the left of the mesenteric vessels is distal pancreatectomy
(C) management of a ductal injury to the right of the mesenteric vessels is pancreaticoduodenectomy
(D) fistulas that result from drainage of pancreatic injuries nearly always heal spontaneously
(E) small peripancreatic hematomas should be explored to search for pancreatic injury

Questions 132–133

132. A 27-year-old woman is brought to the emergency room for evaluation after her car crashes into a tree. Vital signs are stable. She has generalized abdominal pain but no peritoneal signs or respiratory distress. There is a small amount of blood returning from the nasogastric tube. Chest x-rays and a Gastrografin swallow are shown below. The patient should be prepared for which of the following procedures?

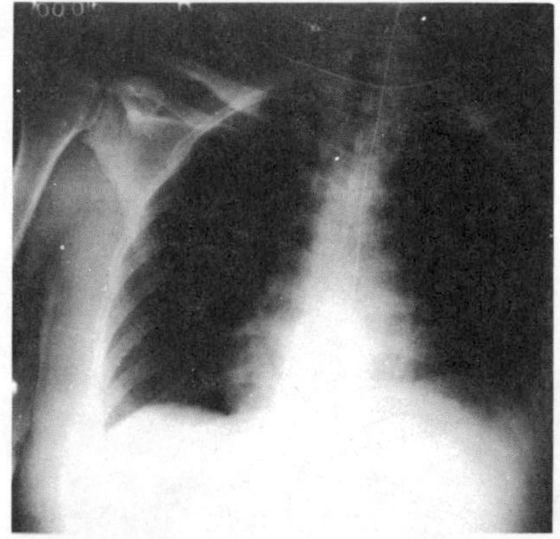

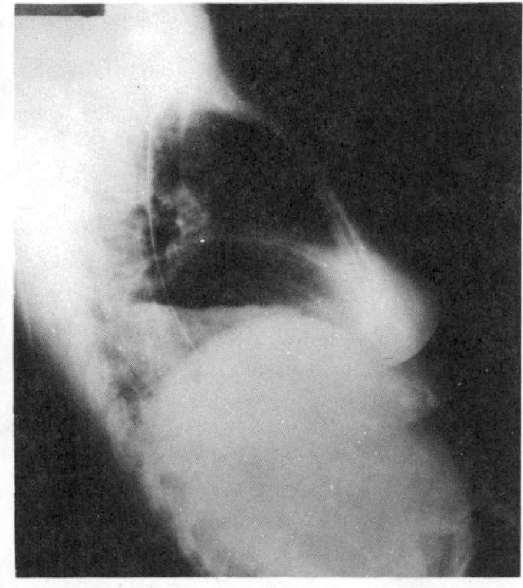

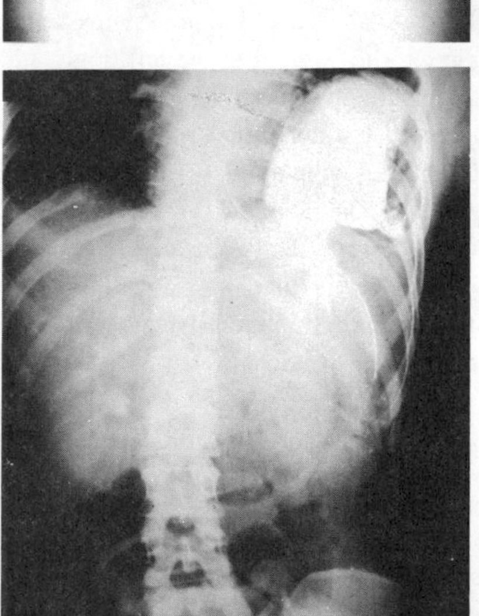

(A) Celiotomy
(B) Left thoracotomy
(C) Bronchoscopy
(D) Chest tube insertion into the left intrapleural space
(E) Continuous nasogastric tube suction and observation

133. All the following statements about the previously described injury are correct EXCEPT that

(A) a similar injury on the right side is uncommon
(B) related signs and symptoms may not develop for months or years following injury
(C) acute respiratory insufficiency may develop
(D) urgent surgical treatment is indicated
(E) nonsurgical management is indicated in the asymptomatic patient

134. Which of the following abdominal lesions is LEAST likely to follow a rapid deceleration injury?

(A) Renal vascular injury
(B) Superior mesenteric thrombosis
(C) Mesenteric vascular injury
(D) Avulsion of the splenic pedicle
(E) Diaphragmatic hernia

135. Blunt trauma to the abdomen most commonly injures which of the following organs?

(A) Liver
(B) Kidney
(C) Spleen
(D) Intestine
(E) Pancreas

136. Repair of injured peripheral veins is preferable to ligation for all the following reasons EXCEPT that

(A) in popliteal injuries, ligation leads to an increased amputation rate despite successful arterial reconstruction
(B) ligation leads to an increased incidence of chronic venous insufficiency
(C) ligation leads to an increased incidence of pulmonary embolization
(D) in the presence of extensive associated soft tissue injury, venous return already is significantly impaired
(E) even though repaired veins thrombose, they often recanalize

137. A 27-year-old man sustains a single gunshot wound to the left thigh. In the emergency room he is noted to have a large hematoma of his medial thigh. He complains of paresthesias in his foot. On examination there are weak pulses palpable distal to the injury and he is unable to move his foot. The appropriate initial management of this patient would be

(A) angiography
(B) immediate exploration and repair
(C) fasciotomy of anterior compartment
(D) observation for resolution of spasm
(E) local wound exploration

Questions 138–139

A 25-year-old woman arrives in the emergency room following an automobile accident. She is acutely dyspneic with a respiratory rate of 60/min. Breath sounds are markedly diminished on the right side.

138. The first step in managing the patient should be to

(A) take a chest x-ray
(B) draw arterial blood for blood gas determination
(C) decompress the right pleural space
(D) perform pericardiocentesis
(E) administer intravenous fluids

139. A chest x-ray of this woman before therapy would probably reveal all the following EXCEPT

(A) air in the right pleural space
(B) shifting of the mediastinum toward the left
(C) compression of the left lung
(D) shifting of the trachea toward the left
(E) fluid in the left pleural cavity

140. The management of a complete transection of the common bile duct distal to the insertion of the cystic duct may include all the following EXCEPT

(A) ligation of the common duct, cholecystojejunostomy
(B) loop choledochojejunostomy
(C) primary end-to-end anastomosis
(D) Roux en Y choledochojejunostomy
(E) bridging the injury with a T-tube

141. Although nonoperative management of penetrating neck injuries has been advocated as an alternative to mandatory exploration in asymptomatic patients, all the following findings would necessitate formal neck exploration EXCEPT

(A) expanding hematoma
(B) dysphagia
(C) dysphonia
(D) pneumothorax
(E) hemoptysis

142. Following blunt abdominal trauma, a 12-year-old girl develops upper abdominal pain, nausea, and vomiting. An upper gastrointestinal series reveals a total obstruction of the duodenum with a "coiled spring" appearance in the second and third portions. Appropriate management is

(A) gastrojejunostomy
(B) nasogastric suction and observation
(C) duodenal resection
(D) TPN to increase size of retroperitoneal fat pad
(E) duodenojejunostomy

DIRECTIONS: Each question below contains four suggested responses of which **one or more** is correct. Select

A	if	**1, 2, and 3**	are correct
B	if	**1 and 3**	are correct
C	if	**2 and 4**	are correct
D	if	**4**	is correct
E	if	**1, 2, 3, and 4**	are correct

143. A 26-year-old man sustains a gunshot wound to the left thigh. Exploration reveals that a 2-cm portion of superficial femoral artery is destroyed. Appropriate management may include

(1) debridement and end-to-end anastomosis
(2) debridement and repair with interposition gortex graft
(3) debridement and repair with interposition vein graft
(4) ligation and observation

144. A 36-year-old man sustains a gunshot wound to the left buttock. He is hemodynamically stable. There is no exit wound and an x-ray of the abdomen shows the bullet to be located in the right lower quadrant. Proctoscopic examination in the emergency room reveals fresh blood and clots in the rectal ampulla and a through and through injury to the rectum at 6 cm from the anal verge. Appropriate management would include

(1) diverting colostomy
(2) irrigation of distal rectum
(3) debridement and closure of rectal injuries
(4) presacral drainage

145. Correct statements regarding blunt trauma to the liver include which of the following?

(1) Hepatic artery ligation for control of bleeding is associated with decreased morbidity and mortality
(2) The incidence of intraabdominal infections is significantly lower in patients with abdominal drains
(3) Intracaval shunting has dramatically improved survival among patients with hepatic vein injuries
(4) Nonanatomic hepatic debridement, with removal of the injured fragments only, is preferable to resection along anatomic planes

146. If traumatic injury to an artery in a major extremity is suspected by clinical or angiographic examination, surgical exploration should be carried out regardless of the presence of palpable pulses distal to the injury. The rationale for this procedure includes which of the following statements?

(1) Subsequent development of arteriovenous fistulae and false aneurysms can be avoided
(2) The presence of palpable distal pulses does not reliably exclude significant arterial trauma
(3) Intimal injuries can lead to delayed arterial occlusion
(4) Prophylactic fasciotomy should be performed to avert an anterior compartment syndrome

147. The response to shock includes which of the following metabolic effects?

(1) Sodium and water retention
(2) Shift to anaerobic metabolism
(3) Hyperkalemia
(4) Hyperglycemia

148. Correct statements concerning traumatic diaphragmatic hernia include which of the following?

(1) Strangulation of abdominal viscera may complicate the herniation
(2) The peripheral muscular portion of the diaphragm is usually affected
(3) Bowel sounds may be heard upon auscultation of the chest
(4) Most traumatic diaphragmatic hernias occur on the right side

149. Appropriate treatment for an acute stable hematoma of the pinna of the ear includes which of the following measures?

(1) Ice packs and prophylactic antibiotics
(2) Excision of the hematoma
(3) Needle aspiration
(4) Incision, drainage, and pressure bandage

150. Animal and clinical studies have shown that administration of lactated Ringer's solution to patients with hypovolemic shock may

(1) decrease serum lactate concentration
(2) avert the need for transfusion of whole blood
(3) improve hemodynamics by alleviating the deficit in the interstitial fluid compartment
(4) increase metabolic acidosis

151. During celiotomy for blunt trauma with associated pelvic fractures, a large pelvic retroperitoneal hematoma is discovered. The patient receives 6 units of blood during the procedure and is hemodynamically stable. There are no other significant intraabdominal injuries. Management of this hematoma should include

(1) exploration and ligation of both internal iliac arteries
(2) observation of hematoma and no further therapy if it is not expanding
(3) packing of the pelvis for 24 to 80 hours to aid in tamponade
(4) postoperative angiography to rule out major vascular injury

SUMMARY OF DIRECTIONS

A	B	C	D	E
1,2,3 only	1,3 only	2,4 only	4 only	All are correct

Questions 152–153

An 18-year-old high school football player is kicked in the left flank. Three hours later he develops hematuria. His vital signs are stable.

152. Initial diagnostic tests in the emergency room should include which of the following?

(1) Retrograde urethrography
(2) Retrograde cystography
(3) Arteriography
(4) High-dose infusion urography

153. The diagnostic tests performed reveal extravasation of contrast into the renal parenchyma. Treatment should consist of

(1) Increased fluid intake and antibiotics
(2) exploration and suture of laceration
(3) serial monitoring of blood count and vital signs
(4) nephrostomy

154. True statements regarding tendon injuries in the hand include which of the following?

(1) Flexor digitorum superficialis inserts on the middle phalanx
(2) Flexor digitorum profundus inserts on the distal phalanx
(3) The tendons of flexor digitorum profundus arise from a common muscle belly
(4) The best results for repair of a flexor tendon are obtained with injuries in the fibroosseous tunnel (zone 2)

DIRECTIONS: Each group of questions below consists of four lettered headings followed by a set of numbered items. For each numbered item select

A	if the item is associated with	(A) **only**
B	if the item is associated with	(B) **only**
C	if the item is associated with	**both** (A) and (B)
D	if the item is associated with	**neither** (A) nor (B)

Each lettered heading may be used **once, more than once, or not at all.**

Questions 155–158

(A) Peritoneal lavage
(B) Computed abdominal tomography
(C) Both
(D) Neither

155. Useful in evaluating retroperitoneal injury

156. Useful in evaluating intraperitoneal injury

157. Useful in obtaining hemostasis in lieu of laparotomy

158. Useful in detecting as little as 20 ml of intraperitoneal blood

Questions 159–163

(A) Acute splenic rupture
(B) Acute duodenal rupture
(C) Both
(D) Neither

159. Symptoms frequently arise 2 to 4 days later

160. Celiotomy is necessary once the diagnosis is made

161. Upper GI series may show a "coil spring" intestinal pattern

162. Peritoneal lavage is usually diagnostic in equivocal cases

163. Signs and symptoms of hemorrhage usually occur within hours

DIRECTIONS: Each group of questions below consists of lettered headings followed by a set of numbered items. For each numbered item select the **one** lettered heading with which it is **most** closely associated. Each lettered heading may be used **once, more than once, or not at all.**

Questions 164–168

For each of the immediately life-threatening injuries of the chest listed below, select the proper intervention.

(A) Endotracheal intubation
(B) Cricothyroidotomy
(C) Subxiphoid window
(D) Tube thoracostomy
(E) Occlusive dressing

164. Airway obstruction

165. Open pneumothorax

166. Flail chest

167. Tension pneumothorax

168. Pericardial tamponade

Questions 169–172

For each of the following case histories, select the most appropriate diagnostic procedure.

(A) Angiography
(B) Computerized tomography
(C) Ultrasonography
(D) Surgical exploration
(E) Peritoneal lavage

169. A 35-year-old diabetic man sustains a stab wound of the left midabdomen. Vital signs are normal. Local exploration of the wound reveals penetration beyond the peritoneum

170. A 46-year-old woman has been hit over the occipital skull with a pipe. As she is being evaluated, she develops an enlarging right pupil and becomes progressively lethargic

171. A 21-year-old man traveling in a car at 35 miles an hour collides with a stationary car and strikes his chest against the steering wheel. In the emergency room his vital signs and physical examination are normal. Chest x-ray reveals a widened mediastinum

172. An inebriated 45-year-old man falls down two flights of stairs. On examination he is alternately agitated and stuporous. There are superficial lacerations of the scalp but no other evidence of trauma. Blood pressure is 90/60 mmHg, pulse 120/min, hematocrit 32%. Chest, abdominal, pelvic, and extremity x-rays are negative

Trauma and Shock Answers

119. The answer is D. *(Schwartz, ed 5. pp 271–273.)* The spleen should be salvaged in children if at all possible because of the postsplenectomy septicemia seen at a significantly increased rate in this group. The organisms responsible are most frequently *Diplococcus pneumoniae* and *Haemophilus influenzae*. The most effective method of spleen salvage is via suture repair of the injured segment (splenorrhaphy).

120. The answer is A. *(Shoemaker, p 892. Wilson, Surg Clin North Am 57:17–35, 1977.)* The preeminent concern in treatment of rib fractures is the prevention of pulmonary complications (atelectasis and pneumonia), particularly for patients with preexisting pulmonary disease, who are in danger of progressing to respiratory failure. Attempts to relieve pain by immobilization or splinting, such as strapping the chest, merely compound the problem of inadequate ventilation. Mild pain may be controlled with oral analgesics, and patients with minor fracture injuries, if they can be closely monitored, may be managed at home with appropriate instructions for coughing and deep breathing. Patients with significant fractures or severe pain should be hospitalized. Rib fractures in the elderly are particularly treacherous. Intercostal nerve blocks often provide prolonged periods of pain relief and, together with appropriate pulmonary physiotherapy, will inhibit development of respiratory complications. Rib fractures are often associated with either intrathoracic or intraabdominal injuries. In particular, fractures of the left chest wall should arouse suspicion of splenic trauma. In equivocal cases, abdominal paracentesis will often be diagnostic.

121. The answer is B. *(Schwartz, ed 5. pp 1845–1847. Shires, ed 3. pp 257–263.)* Transection of a peripheral nerve results in hemorrhage and in retraction of the severed nerve ends. Almost immediately, degeneration of the axon distal to the injury begins. Degeneration also occurs in the proximal fragment back to the first node of Ranvier. Phagocytosis of the degenerated axonal fragments leaves a neurilemmal sheath with empty cylindrical spaces where the axons had been. Several days following the injury, axons from the proximal fragment begin to regrow. If they make contact with the distal neurilemmal sheath, regrowth occurs at about the rate of 1 mm per day. However, if associated trauma, fracture, infection, or separation of neurilemmal sheath ends precludes contact between axons, growth is haphazard and a traumatic neuroma is formed. When neural transection is associated with widespread soft tissue damage and hemorrhage (with increased probability of infection), many surgeons choose to delay reapproximation of the severed nerve end for 3 to 4 weeks.

122. The answer is B. *(Shires, ed 3. pp 270–272.)* The young woman presented in the question was admitted to the hospital with small bowel obstruction associated with a chronic diaphragmatic hernia resulting from a seat belt injury 4 years previously. The x-rays shown in the question revealed dilated and air-filled bowel in the chest initially; a subsequent upper GI series demonstrated that the hernia contained loops of jejunum. Acute rupture of the diaphragm caused by blunt or penetrating trauma should be repaired via an abdominal approach, which allows identification and management of associated injuries. In a case of chronic diaphragmatic rupture, a thoracic approach facilitates repair because of the likelihood that serious adhesions to the lung exist. Such hernias have no sac (pleural or peritoneal) and the visceral serosal surfaces of the lung and gut often are intimately fused; they cannot be safely approached from the abdomen. The thoracoabdominal incision (in which the costochondral junction is divided) gives excellent exposure but is an extremely disabling procedure for the patient and has a very high postoperative complication rate; it is rarely justified. Even large defects in the diaphragm can be repaired directly, although occasionally reimplantation into the chest wall at a higher level may be necessary. During the period following rupture (or laceration) of the diaphragm, the persisting negative pressure in the pleural space will cause migration of abdominal contents into the chest and thus gradual enlargement of even very small defects. This pressure differential between chest and abdomen greatly increases the likelihood of eventual incarceration of the bowel and significant loss of lung volume. Therefore, injuries to the diaphragm should be repaired as soon as they are diagnosed, since the complications may be life threatening. This patient is sucking air and intestinal juice into the intrathoracic portion of her intestine with each respiratory effort. Although passage of a nasogastric tube relieves dilatation of the stomach during periods of acute distress and remarkable improvement in symptoms may occur, the patient remains at high risk until the defect has been surgically corrected.

123–126. The answers are: 123-A, 124-E, 125-B, 126-B. *(Shires, ed 3. pp 232–236. Walt, ed 3. pp 184–190.)* Closed head injuries may result in cerebral concussion from depression of the reticular formation of the brainstem. This type of injury is usually reversible.

Local bleeding and swelling (intracranial or extracranial) produce an increase in the intracranial pressure. A characteristic symptom pattern occurs initiated by progressive depression of mental status. Increasing intracranial pressure tends to displace brain tissue away from the source of the pressure; if the pressure is sufficient, herniation of the uncal process through the tentorium cerebri occurs.

Pupillary dilatation is caused by compression of the ipsilateral oculomotor nerve and its parasympathetic fibers. If the pressure is not relieved, the contralateral oculomotor nerve will become involved and, ultimately, the brainstem herniates through the foramen magnum, causing death. Hypertension and bradycardia are preterminal events.

Emergency measures to reduce intracranial pressure while preparing for localization of the clot or for a craniotomy or both include hyperventilation, dexamethasone (Decadron), and mannitol infusion. Of these, hyperventilation produces the most rapid decrease in brain swelling.

127. The answer is A. *(Hardy, ed 2. pp 166–171.)* Flail chest is diagnosed in the presence of paradoxical respiratory movement in a portion of the chest wall. At least two fractures in each of three adjacent ribs or costal cartilages are required to produce this condition. Complications of flail chest include segmental pulmonary hypoventilation with subsequent infection and ultimately respiratory failure. Management of flail chest should be individualized. If adequate pain control and pulmonary toilet can be provided, patients may be managed without stabilization of the flail. Often intercostal nerve blocks and tracheostomy aid in this form of management. If stabilization is required, external methods such as sandbags or towel clips are no longer used. Surgical stabilization with wires is used if thoracotomy is to be performed for another indication. If this is not the case, "internal" stabilization is performed by placing the patient on mechanical ventilation with positive end-expiratory pressure. Tracheostomy is recommended because these patients usually require 10 to 14 days to stabilize their flail segment and postventilation pulmonary toilet is simplified by tracheostomy. Indications for mechanical ventilation include significant impedance to ventilation by the flail segment, large pulmonary contusion, an uncooperative patient (e.g., owing to head injury), general anesthesia for another indication, greater than five ribs fractured, and the development of respiratory failure.

128. The answer is D. *(Wilson, Surg Clin North Am 57:17–35, 1977. Zuidema, ed 4. pp 16–17, 423–425.)* Pulmonary contusions are the result of trauma to the lung parenchyma, which is generally caused by rapid-deceleration injury. Opacification seen on chest x-ray is usually localized and develops within minutes of injury, but may then progress over the next 48 to 72 hours. Since the pathophysiological consequences of the injury result from fluid sequestration through damaged capillaries, fluids should be administered sparingly and diuretics used judiciously. Many affected patients require assisted ventilation. With proper treatment, contusions usually resolve in 2 to 5 days.

129. The answer is D. *(Schwartz, ed 5. pp 248–250.)* Gunshot wounds to the lower chest are often associated with intraabdominal injuries. The diaphragm can rise to the level of T4 during maximal expiration. Therefore, any patient with a gunshot wound below the level of T4 should be subjected to abdominal exploration. Exploratory thoracotomy is not indicated because most parenchymal lung injuries will stop bleeding and heal spontaneously with the use of tube thoracostomy alone. Indication for thoracic exploration for bleeding is usually in the range of 100 to 150 ml/hr over several hours. Peritoneal lavage is not indicated even though the abdominal examination is unremarkable. As many as 25 percent of patients with negative physical findings and negative peritoneal lavage will have significant intraabdominal injuries in this setting. These injuries include damage to the colon, kidney, pancreas, aorta, and diaphragm. For similar reasons local wound exploration is not recommended as the determination of diaphragmatic injury with this technique is unreliable.

130. The answer is A. *(Shires, ed 3. p 241.)* Even in the absence of hypovolemic shock, patients who have experienced transection of the cervical cord may present with mild hypotension and bradycardia. While higher cervical transection will cause immediate respiratory failure, lower cervical transection may be followed within hours by ascending cord edema and consequent respiratory compromise. Cord interruption leads to an initial flaccid paralysis and loss of all deep tendon reflexes. Later in the course a spastic paralysis and hyperreflexic state may develop. Owing to loss of autonomic function and inability to sweat, hyperthermia may develop.

131. The answer is C. *(Schwartz, ed 5. pp 267–271.)* The majority of penetrating pancreatic injuries can be managed with simple drainage. When a pancreatic fistula develops it is usually minor and closes within 1 month. Prolonged drainage on high-output fistulas also will usually heal spontaneously but may require the institution of TPN in order to provide adequate nutrition to stimulate healing as well as decreasing pancreatic secretions. Injury to the major pancreatic duct to the left of the mesenteric vessels is effectively treated with a distal pancreatectomy. The high morbidity and mortality of a pancreaticoduodenectomy for trauma limit its use to extensive blunt injuries to both pancreatic head and duodenum. For ductal injury in the region of the head of the pancreas a Roux en Y limb of jejunum should be brought up and used to drain the transected duct. The proximity of the pancreas to many other major structures makes combined injuries frequent (90 percent). Complications of pancreatic injury include fistula, pseudocyst, and abscess, but the cause of death in patients with pancreatic injury is most frequently exsanguination from associated injury to major vascular structures such as the splenic vessels, mesenteric vessels, aorta, or inferior vena cava. Finally, however small, all peripancreatic hematomas should be explored to search for pancreatic injury. Simple drainage is usually adequate treatment in such cases but failure to recognize a pancreatic injury can have catastrophic sequelae.

132–133. The answers are: 132-A, 133-E. *(Wilson, Surg Clin North Am 57:17–35, 1977.)* The films depicted in the question are diagnostic of traumatic rupture of the left diaphragm with intrathoracic herniation of the stomach. Urgent surgical repair is indicated to prevent gastric obstruction and strangulation and to preclude development of respiratory failure. While transthoracic repair is recommended if the diagnosis is delayed beyond several weeks or if the hernia is on the right side, the acute injury is appropriately approached transabdominally to assess for associated injuries, which are present in approximately 75 percent of affected patients.

Almost 90 percent of diaphragmatic injuries following blunt trauma occur on the left, probably because of the protective effect of the liver on the right side. Related signs and symptoms are absent in about one third of patients. Diaphragmatic injury should be suspected if plain films reveal abnormal densities in the left lower lung field, if the diaphragmatic outline is obscured or elevated, or if the mediastinum is shifted to the right. Gastrointestinal contrast studies will usually confirm the diagnosis.

134. The answer is E. *(Sabiston, ed 13. pp 400–407. Shires, ed 3. pp 291–340.)* In the rapid-deceleration injury associated with automobile crashes, the abdominal viscera tend to continue moving anteriorly after the body wall has been stopped. These organs exert great stress upon the structures anchoring them to the retroperitoneum. Intestinal loops stretch and may tear their mesenteric attachments, injuring and thrombosing the superior mesenteric artery; kidneys and spleen may similarly shear their vascular pedicles. In these injuries, however, ordinarily the intraabdominal pressure does not rise excessively and diaphragmatic hernia is not likely. Diaphragmatic hernia is primarily associated with compression-type abdominal or thoracic injuries that increase intraabdominal or intrathoracic pressure sufficiently to tear the central portion of the diaphragm.

135. The answer is C. *(Schwartz, ed 5. pp 243–278. Shires, ed 3. pp 291–340. Walt, ed 3. pp 142–159.)* The diagnosis of injuries resulting from blunt abdominal trauma is difficult; injuries often are masked by associated injuries. Thus, trauma to the head or chest, together with fractures, frequently conceals intraabdominal injury. Apparently trivial injuries may rupture abdominal viscera in spite of the protection offered by the rib cage. The structures most likely to be damaged in blunt abdominal trauma are, in order of frequency, spleen, kidney, intestine, liver, abdominal wall, mesentery, pancreas, and diaphragm. Abdominal paracentesis is a rapid, sensitive diagnostic test for patients with suspected intraabdominal injury and may be extremely helpful in the management of patients with associated head, thoracic, or pelvic trauma in whom signs and symptoms of the abdominal injuries may be masked or overlooked.

136. The answer is C. *(Zuidema, ed 4. pp 631–655.)* Ligation rather than repair of large veins in the extremities has, in the past, been advocated in patients with multiple injuries or severe trauma. Venous repair adds to the operative time, often results in thrombosis and occlusion, and was thought to lead to an increased incidence of pulmonary embolization. Recent studies, including reviews of the Viet Nam Vascular Registry, indicate that the risk of pulmonary embolization is *not* increased with repair and that vein repair, in conjunction with arterial repair, increases limb salvage, particularly in popliteal injuries. Venous repair may also be necessary in the presence of extensive soft tissue trauma and an already severely compromised venous return. Long-term follow-up reveals that the sequelae of chronic venous insufficiency are developing with increasing frequency in those patients who have had lower extremity vein ligations. Morbidity from chronic deep venous occlusion may be diminished even in those patients who develop thrombosis following repair, since recanalization often occurs. For these reasons, it is currently recommended that large veins be repaired whenever clinically feasible.

137. The answer is B. *(Schwartz, ed 5. p 947.)* The five *p*'s of arterial injury include pain, paresthesias, pallor, pulselessness, and paralysis. The most sensitive tissues in the extremity to anoxia are the peripheral nerves and striated muscle. The early developments of paresthesias and paralysis are signals that there is significant ischemia present and immediate exploration and repair are warranted. The presence of palpable pulses does not exclude an arterial injury as this presence may represent a transmitted pulsation through a blood clot. When severe ischemia is present the repair must be completed within 6 to 8 hours to prevent irreversible muscle ischemia and loss of limb function. Delay to obtain an angiogram or to observe for change needlessly prolongs the ischemic time. Fasciotomy may be required but should be done in conjunction with and after reestablishment of arterial flow. Local wound exploration is not recommended because brisk hemorrhage may be encountered without the securing of prior vascular control.

138–139. The answers are: 138-C, 139-E. *(Hardy, ed 2. pp 166–171. Wiot JAMA 231:500–503, 1975.)* Tension pneumothorax is a life-threatening problem requiring immediate treatment. A lung wound that behaves as a ball or flap valve allows escaped air to build up pressure in the intrapleural space. This causes collapse of the ipsilateral lung and shifting of the mediastinum and trachea to the contralateral side, in addition to compression of the vena cava and contralateral lung. Sudden death may ensue because of a decrease in the cardiac output, hypoxemia, and ventricular arrhythmias. To accomplish rapid decompression of the pleural space, a large-gauge needle should be passed into the intrapleural cavity through the second intercostal space at the midclavicular line. This may be attached temporarily to an underwater seal with subsequent insertion of a chest tube after the life-threatening urgency has been relieved.

Tension pneumothorax produces characteristic x-ray findings of ipsilateral lung collapse, mediastinal and tracheal shift, and compression of the contralateral lung. Occasionally, adhesions prevent complete lung collapse, but the tension pneumothorax is evident because of the mediastinal displacement. A pleural effusion would not be expected acutely in the absence of associated intrapleural blood.

140. The answer is C. *(Schwartz, ed 5. pp 264–266.)* Traumatic injury to the common bile duct must be considered in two separate categories. Complete transection of the common bile duct can be handled in many ways. If the patient is unstable and time is limited, simply placing a T-tube in either end of the open common bile duct and staging the repair is the treatment of choice. In a stable patient a biliary enteric bypass is preferred. This can be accomplished by Roux en Y choledochojejunostomy or cholecystojejunostomy. The jejunum is favored over the duodenum because if the anastomosis leaks a lateral duodenal fistula is avoided. For similar reasons the defunctionalization of the jejunal limb is also preferable. This can be accomplished by creating a Roux en Y limb or by performing an enteroenterostomy distal to an anastomosis created with a loop of jejunum. Primary end-to-end repair of a completely transected common bile duct is not recommended because of the high incidence of stricture and need for reoperation and creation of a biliary enteric bypass. However, end-to-end repair is the procedure of choice if the common bile duct is lacerated or only partially transected.

141. The answer is D. *(Davis, pp 2768–2821.)* Reports of a more than 50 percent incidence of negative explorations of the neck, iatrogenic complications, and serious injuries overlooked at operation have caused a reassessment of the dictum that all penetrating neck wounds that violate the platysma must be explored. Stable patients with high (zone III) or low (zone I) injuries, or multiple neck wounds, should undergo initial angiography irrespective of their ultimate treatment plan. Algorithms exist for nonoperative management of asymptomatic patients, employing observation alone, or combinations of vascular and aerodigestive contrast studies and endoscopy. Nevertheless, recognition of acute signs of airway distress (stridor, hoarseness, dysphonia), visceral injury (subcutaneous air, hemoptysis, dysphagia), hemorrhage (expanding hematoma, unchecked external bleeding), or neurologic symptoms referable to carotid injury (stroke or altered mental status) or lower cranial nerve or brachial plexus injury requires formal neck exploration. Pneumothorax would mandate a chest tube; the necessity for exploration, additional studies (such as angiography, in a stable zone I injury), or observation alone would depend on clinical judgment and institutional policy.

142. The answer is B. *(Schwartz, ed 5. p 256.)* Duodenal hematomas result from blunt abdominal trauma. They present as a high bowel obstruction with abdominal pain and occasionally a palpable right upper quadrant mass. An upper gastrointestinal series is almost diagnostic with the classic coiled spring appearance of the second and third portions of the duodenum secondary to the crowding of the valvulae conniventes (circular folds) by the hematoma. Nonsurgical management is the mainstay of therapy as the vast majority of duodenal hematomas resolve spontaneously. Simple evacuation of the hematoma is the operative procedure of choice. However, bypass procedures and duodenal resection have been performed for this problem. In patients with duodenal obstruction from the superior mesenteric artery syndrome, the obstruction is usually the result of a marked weight loss and, in conjunction with this, loss of the retroperitoneal fat pad that elevates the superior mesenteric artery from the third and fourth portions of the duodenum. Nutritional repletion and replenishment of this fat pad will elevate the artery off the duodenum and relieve the obstruction.

143. The answer is B (1, 3). *(Schwartz, ed 5. p 938.)* Traumatic arterial injuries can be handled with several techniques. The basic principles of debridement of injured tissue and reestablishment of flow should be observed. Primary end-to-end anastomosis is preferable if this can be accomplished without tension. When 2 cm of artery has been destroyed it is often not possible to perform a tension-free primary anastomosis. In this case a reversed saphenous vein graft is the repair of choice. Ligation of the artery is to be avoided in order to avoid gangrene and limb loss. The use of prosthetic material (gortex) in a potentially infected field is also to be avoided as infection at the suture line often leads to delayed hemorrhage.

144. The answer is E (all). *(Schwartz, ed 5. p 259.)* Traumatic perforations of the extraperitoneal rectum can lead to devastating infectious complications if mishandled. The principles of management are similar to those for intraperitoneal injuries to the large intestine; that is, the wound should be debrided and closed if easily accessible. In all cases of rectal injury a diverting colostomy and presacral drainage are mandatory. Failure to accomplish fecal diversion and drainage can result in perineal sepsis, which can spread through fascial planes involving the lower extremities and trunk with devastating consequences. Finally, irrigation of the distal rectum to remove fecal material is often advocated to maintain low rates of infectious complications.

145. The answer is D (4). *(Cox, Ann Surg 207:126–134, 1988.)* The overwhelming majority of patients explored for blunt trauma to the liver sustain their injuries in motor vehicle accidents. In a large consecutive series of patients (n = 323) with blunt hepatic trauma who were explored for the finding of hemoperitoneum on peritoneal lavage, the mortality was 31 percent. Forty-two percent of the deaths, due primarily to liver injury, occurred intraoperatively during the initial operation following admission. All operations were performed at a regional trauma center by staff trauma surgeons. Their findings included the following observations: (1) intraoperative deaths were due to uncontrolled hemorrhage; (2) patients with major hepatic injuries who survived operation but nevertheless died appeared to succumb either to sepsis or to associated injuries, usually involving the head or chest; (3) hepatic artery ligation for control of bleeding yielded dismal results; of the three surviving patients who underwent hepatic artery ligation (an additional 11 died), two required reoperation for continued bleeding; (4) the use of drains (passive and active) was associated with a significantly greater incidence of intraabdominal infectious complications; (5) intracaval shunting was used in 7 severely injured patients without a survivor; (6) while minor hepatic injuries required little or no treatment, major lacerations could usually be controlled with simple absorbable sutures placed 2 to 3 cm from the fracture edge, without occurrence of subsequent intrahepatic hematomata, hemobilia, or bile fistulae; (7) hepatic fragmentation may be treated by nonanatomic debridement, with suture ligation of individual bleeding points; of nine attempts at formal anatomic resection in stable patients, all ended in uncontrollable hemorrhage and death.

146. The answer is A (1, 2, 3). *(Zuidema, ed 4. pp 631–636).* The presence of ischemic changes following vascular trauma is an indication for emergency exploration and repair. Nonsurgical management of arterial trauma when distal pulses are palpable may lead to delayed sequelae of embolization, occlusion, secondary hemorrhage, false aneurysm, and traumatic arteriovenous fistula. The presence of palpable pulses does not reliably exclude significant arterial injury. Injuries that may be missed if exploration is not performed include lacerations and partial transections containing hematomas, intramural or intraluminal thromboses, and intimal disruptions or tears. Prophylactic fasciotomy is not routinely performed for all arterial injuries but is indicated in the presence of an ischemic period exceeding 4 to 6 hours, combined arterial and major venous injury, prolonged periods of hypotension, massive associated soft tissue trauma, and massive edema.

147. The answer is E (all). *(Hardy, ed 2. pp 36–38.)* The biochemical changes associated with shock result from tissue hypoperfusion, endocrine response to stress, and specific organ system failure. During shock, the sympathetic nervous system and adrenal medulla are stimulated to release catecholamines. Renin, angiotensin, antidiuretic hormone, adrenocorticotropin, and cortisol levels increase. Resultant changes include sodium and water retention, increase in potassium excretion, protein catabolism, and gluconeogenesis. Potassium levels rise as a result of increased tissue release, anaerobic metabolism, and decreased renal perfusion. If renal function is maintained, potassium excretion is high and normal plasma potassium levels are restored.

148. The answer is B (1, 3). *(Schwartz, ed 5. p 649.)* Blunt abdominal or thoracic trauma may rupture the diaphragm as a result of increasing abdominal or thoracic pressure. Generally, the central or tendinous portion of the diaphragm is torn. Almost all ruptures occur on the left side, as the liver seems to guard the right side against rupture. Abdominal viscera may extend through the defect into the pleural space, leading to pulmonary compression and respiratory distress or to intestinal obstruction and possible strangulation. Bowel sounds frequently may be heard upon auscultation of the chest. Operative repair of a diaphragmatic hernia is indicated as soon as the patient's general condition permits.

149. The answer is D (4). *(Sabiston, ed 13. pp 1403–1404.)* A subperichondrial hematoma in the pinna of the ear may lead to avascular necrosis of the cartilage with shriveling of the pinna and fibrosis and calcification of the hematoma. The result is the deformity known as "cauliflower ear." Appropriate treatment consists of evacuation of the hematoma by incision and tight packing of the skin and perichondrium onto the cartilage with a pressure dressing. Needle aspiration does not effect adequate drainage. Ice packs may be helpful early, but are not sufficient to prevent the deformity; antibiotics are not indicated for this lesion. Since the hematoma is subperichondrial, excision of the hematoma would remove the perichondrium and lead to cartilage deformities.

150. The answer is A (1, 2, 3). *(Schwartz, ed 5. p 218. Shires, ed 3. pp 16–17.)* Infusion of lactated Ringer's solution is an effective immediate step, both clinically and experimentally, in managing hypovolemic shock. Use of this balanced salt solution helps correct the fluid deficit (in the extracellular, extravascular compartment) resulting from hypovolemic shock. This procedure may decrease requirements for whole blood in patients with hemorrhagic shock. If blood loss has been minimal and is controlled, whole blood transfusion may be avoided entirely. The theoretic objection to infusion of lactated Ringer's solution is that it will increase lactate levels and compound the problem of lactic acidosis. This has not been borne out in animal or clinical studies. Along with the hemodynamic improvement that follows volume restitution, liver function improves, lactate metabolism is improved, excess lactate levels drop, and metabolic acidosis improves.

151. The answer is C (2, 4). *(Schwartz, ed 5. pp 273–274.)* The management of retroperitoneal hematomas is generally aggressive with exploration of all such hematomas in order not to miss major vascular or visceral injuries. The exception to this rule is the pelvic retroperitoneal hematoma that develops after pelvic fractures. These hematomas can be quite significant with as much as 2 to 4 L of blood being sequestered in this region. However, spontaneous tamponade usually occurs. If these hematomas are explored, hemorrhage from multiple bleeding points that is often impossible to control may result. Therefore, if the size of the hematoma is stable and the patient is hemodynamically stable, it is recommended that these hematomas not be explored. In the case of very large hematomas it is advisable to obtain radiographic evidence that there has been no injury to the major vascular structures of this area (aorta and iliac vessels). Attempts to control hemorrhage from this area are often futile, but when the physician is forced to explore these hematomas because of failure of spontaneous tamponade, techniques advocated include bilateral internal iliac ligation, packing of the pelvis for 24 to 48 hours, and angiographic embolization of pelvic vessels.

152–153. The answers are: 152-D (4), 153-B (1, 3). *(Pontes, Surg Clin North Am 57:77–96, 1977. Zuidema, ed 4. pp 528–534.)* In stable patients with suspected genitourinary tract injury, the first urologic study other than a urinalysis should be the intravenous urogram. The high dose drip infusion technique is desirable because the high concentration of contrast achieved greatly facilitates interpretation in an unprepared patient. Intravenous urography should be performed before retrograde cystography to avoid obscuring visualization of the lower ureteral tract. The study also may preclude the need for retrograde urethrography in patients where, unlike the case presented, there is a suspicion of urethral injury. Renal arteriography is not indicated routinely but should be performed to rule out renal pedicle injury when no kidney function is demonstrated by drip infusion urography.

Seventy to eighty percent of patients with blunt renal trauma are successfully treated nonsurgically. Bed rest may reduce the likelihood of secondary hemorrhage;

antibiotics may reduce the chance of infection's developing in a perirenal hematoma. Failure of conservative treatment is indicated by rising fever, increasing leukocytosis, evidence of secondary hemorrhage, and persistent or increasing pain and tenderness in the region of the kidney.

154. The answer is A (1, 2, 3). *(Schwartz, ed 5. pp 2051–2053.)* Each digit has two long flexors, named superficial and deep according to the relative position of the muscle bellies. In the fingers each superficial flexor tendon divides around the corresponding deep tendon to reach its insertion on the base of the middle phalanx. The deep flexor tendon continues to its insertion on the base of the distal phalanx. Only the deep flexors can flex the distal interphalangeal joint. Since the tendons of the deep flexors share a common muscle belly, only the superficial flexures can move a finger when the adjacent fingers are immobilized. These tendons are prevented from bowstringing across the joints by the flexor retinaculum of the wrist and the fibroosseous tunnels, which extend from the distal palmar crease to the middle phalanx. They run within synovial sheaths and are nourished by vincula tendinum (short mesenteries). The process of healing a tendon injury involves the formation of a tenoma, which tends to become adherent to the surrounding sheath. A difficult balance has to be struck between the desire to prevent adhesions by early mobilization and the risk of rupturing an unhealed tendon. Verdan has divided the hand into six regions according to the anatomy surrounding the tendons. Zone 2 refers to the fibroosseous tunnels. Repair in this region is fraught with difficulty.

155–158. The answers are: 155-B, 156-C, 157-D, 158-A. *(Davis, pp 2789–2790. Walters, Surg Gynecol Obstet 165:496–502, 1988.)* Peritoneal lavage is a diagnostic technique used to identify occult intraperitoneal injury in patients with abdominal trauma. An abnormal lavage is obtained when the lavage effluent exceeds allowable levels of blood, bile, or amylase; the presence of vegetable matter also constitutes an abnormal result. Lavage has been used most widely in the triage of hemodynamically stable victims of abdominal trauma who are suspected of having significant injuries but who manifest equivocal physical findings. Further indications for lavage are the suspicion of abdominal injury in patients with altered sensoria, with unexplained blood loss, and who require general anesthesia to treat other injuries. The technique is exquisitely sensitive to intraabdominal bleeding and will detect as little as 20 ml of free blood in the peritoneal cavity. Because stable retroperitoneal hematomas and minor lacerations of the liver and spleen often shed sufficient blood to produce a positive lavage, some authors have advocated abdominal CT as the preferred method of identifying occult operable injuries of the abdomen. Also, CT with oral and intravenous contrast can provide accurate images of the injured retroperitoneum and the solid intraabdominal viscera (as lavage cannot). Neither CT nor lavage has been a reliable indicator of small intestinal and diaphragmatic injuries; and neither has been useful in obtaining hemostasis nonoperatively. Angiography, however, may be employed to demonstrate visceral or pelvic arterial extravasation and to control hemorrhage by selective embolization.

159–163. The answers are: 159-B, 160-C, 161-D, 162-A, 163-A. *(Schwartz, ed 5. pp 243–278. Shires, ed 3. pp 291–340.)* In blunt trauma, the spleen is the most frequently injured abdominal organ. Although a patient may stabilize temporarily following splenic trauma, progressive signs and symptoms usually develop within hours of the injury. The concept of delayed splenic rupture, reported in the past to occur in 10 to 15 percent of affected persons, more probably represents a delay in proper diagnosis than a distinct syndrome. In equivocal cases, peritoneal lavage is a sensitive test and should yield diagnostic results in over 95 percent of cases. Liver-spleen scans and angiography may be helpful in selected cases of splenic rupture but generally are not necessary; both are costly and invasive procedures. Although much has been written recently about the potential for sepsis following splenectomy, this issue remains unclear, at least in adults; accepted treatment for traumatic splenic injuries remains emergency celiotomy and splenectomy. In selected cases, especially children, in which data supporting postsplenectomy sepsis are most suggestive, attempts to suture peripheral injuries and to control hemorrhage with hemostatic agents appear warranted.

Diagnosing injuries of the duodenum is difficult because of that organ's retroperitoneal location and because duodenal contents are usually sterile and have an almost neutral pH. While symptoms may be delayed for days, early celiotomy is important to survival. Mortality for patients explored 24 hours or more after injury is nearly 40 percent, compared with mortality of only 10 percent for those explored within 24 hours. Aids in the diagnosis of duodenal rupture include plain abdominal

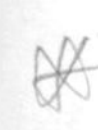

x-rays showing obliteration of the psoas shadow and the presence of retroperitoneal air. Peritoneal lavage may reveal bile, enteric fluid, or an elevated amylase level. When duodenal trauma is suspected, a Gastrografin upper intestinal series should be performed and may demonstrate a site of perforation or rupture. The "coil spring" pattern is characteristic of a submucosal hematoma without perforation.

164–168. The answers are: 164-B, 165-E, 166-A, 167-D, 168-C. *(Hardy, ed 2. pp 166–171. Lawrence, p 140.)* Flail chest describes the paradoxical motion of the chest wall that occurs when consecutive ribs are broken in more than one place, usually following blunt trauma to the thorax. Respiratory distress may ensue when the noncompliant flail segment interferes with generation of adequate positive and negative intrathoracic pressure needed to move air through the trachea. In addition, a blow sufficiently violent to cause a flail chest may also contuse the underlying pulmonary parenchyma, compounding the respiratory distress. Treatment consists of stabilizing the chest wall. Although some temporary benefit may be gained by external buttressing of the chest (e.g., with sandbags, or by turning the patient onto the affected side), endotracheal intubation provides rapid and safe control of the airway, as well as stabilization of the chest internally by positive pressure ventilation.

Airway obstruction denotes partial or complete occlusion of the tracheobronchial tree by foreign bodies, secretions, or crush injuries of the upper respiratory tract. Patients may present with symptoms ranging from cough and mild dyspnea to stridor and hypoxic cardiac arrest. An initial effort should be made to digitally clear the airway and to suction visible secretions; in selected, stable patients, fiberoptic endoscopy may be employed to determine the cause of obstruction and to retrieve foreign objects. Unstable patients whose airways cannot be quickly reestablished by clearing the oropharynx must be intubated. An endotracheal intubation may be attempted, but cricothyroidotomy is indicated in the presence of proximal obstruction or severe maxillofacial trauma.

Blunt or penetrating trauma to the pericardium and heart will result in pericardial tamponade when fluid pressure in the pericardial space exceeds central venous pressure, preventing venous return to the heart. The result is shock, despite adequate volume and myocardial function. The treatment is pericardial decompression. A subxiphoid, supradiaphragmatic incision and creation of a pericardial ''window,'' ideally performed in the operating room, provides a rapid, safe means of confirming the diagnosis of tamponade and of relieving venous obstruction. If heavy bleeding is encountered on opening the pericardial window, a sternotomy may be performed.

Tension pneumothorax occurs when a laceration of the visceral pulmonary pleura acts as a one-way valve, allowing air to enter the pleural space from an underlying parenchymal injury, but not to escape. Increasing intrapleural pressure causes collapse of the ipsilateral lung, compression of the contralateral lung due to mediastinal shift toward the opposite hemithorax, and diminished venous return. Treatment consists of relieving the pneumothorax. This is best accomplished by tube thoracostomy.

Open pneumothorax occurs when a traumatic defect in the chest wall permits free communication of the pleural space with atmospheric pressure. If the defect is larger than two-thirds of the tracheal diameter, respiratory efforts will move air in and out through the defect in the chest wall rather than through the trachea. The immediate treatment is placement of an occlusive dressing over the defect; subsequent interventions include placement of a thoracostomy tube (preferably through a separate incision), formal closure of the chest wall, and ventilatory assistance if needed.

169–172. The answers are: 169-D, 170-B, 171-A, 172-E. *(Fischer, Am Surg 136:701–704, 1978. Schwartz, ed 5. pp 243–278. Shires, ed 3. pp 267–290. Wilson, Surg Clin North Am 57:17–35, 1977.)* Early diagnosis of traumatic rupture of the thoracic aorta is often difficult—there may not be external evidence of chest trauma and tamponading of the injury may mask signs of hemorrhage. Helpful clinical findings include lower extremity pulse deficit, upper extremity hypertension, hoarseness due to pressure on the recurrent laryngeal nerve, and precordial or medial left scapular systolic murmur. Over 90 percent of these injuries occur near the attachment of the ligamentum arteriosum and produce widening of the mediastinum on chest x-ray. This may not be apparent for several hours to several days after injury and repeat films are indicated if the diagnosis of aortic rupture is being considered. Widening of the mediastinum may not reflect aortic injury. Aortography should be performed prior to surgery unless the patient is hemodynamically unstable or the widening mediastinum as shown by x-ray is rapidly progressive.

The patient presented in the last problem is hypotensive with evidence of head trauma but no other obvious signs of injury. The agitation and mental status may reflect inebriation, hypotension, or increased intracranial pressure. The most urgent problem is hypotension, which cannot be presumed secondary to head trauma since intracranial injuries rarely cause a drop in blood pressure. Proper management requires rapid diagnosis and treatment of possible intraperitoneal or retroperitoneal hemorrhage. Peritoneal lavage is a safe, rapid, and highly accurate method for establishing the presence of intraabdominal trauma, with less than 5 percent false positive and false negative results. The value of peritoneal lavage for retroperitoneal injuries, however, is limited. In the event of a negative lavage, the next diagnostic step for this patient might involve intravenous pyelography or angiography or both. A CT scan would be helpful in diagnosis and localization of an intracranial hemorrhage. However, in this patient a CT scan should await hemodynamic stabilization and evaluation of the cause of the hypotension. Celiotomy would be indicated for persistent or progressive shock if a repeat chest x-ray remained normal and pelvic and extremity fractures had been ruled out.

Nonsurgical management of abdominal stab wounds has evolved as appropriate treatment in selected patients. Many negative celiotomies were performed in past years when surgical approach was considered the treatment of choice. Hemodynamically stable patients with small, nonexpanding hematomas, with normal abdominal examination and normal x-ray are safely managed by careful local wound exploration to determine the extent of penetration. If, by this technique, penetration of the peritoneum is documented, celiotomy should be performed. Recent experience with peritoneal lavage suggests that this, too, may be a reliable screening method, particularly for stab wounds at the costal margin or of the back. For patients with injuries proved superficial by these methods, observation rather than surgical exploration is appropriate. Sonography and digital or clamp probing of a wound or tract are unreliable techniques because of changing tissue planes.

Proper surgical management of acute subdural, epidural, and intracerebral hemorrhage requires accurate localization and evacuation of clots and blood by craniotomy. Burr holes are usually inadequate. The time spent in confirming a diagnosis and localizing a hematoma is generally justified and appropriate if emergency CT scanning is available. Exploratory burr holes may be required for those patients with severe multiple injuries as well as for the head trauma victim who requires immediate surgery for thoracoabdominal injuries. Appropriate treatment for the increase in intracranial pressure following head injury includes hyperventilation and administration of dexamethasone and mannitol. These measures can be instituted while awaiting CT scan results and preparing for craniotomy.

Transplants, Immunology, and Oncology

DIRECTIONS: Each question below contains five suggested responses. Select the **one best** response to each question.

173. Cellular immunity to tumor antigens can be demonstrated by all the following EXCEPT

(A) lymphocyte-mediated cytotoxicity
(B) lymphocyte blastogenesis
(C) immunodiffusion
(D) migration inhibition
(E) cutaneous hypersensitivity

174. Death rates from cancer have increased steadily over the past 40 years in primary cancers of the

(A) breast
(B) colon
(C) lung
(D) stomach
(E) uterus

175. Of the surgical procedures listed below, all are useful in the management of non-Hodgkin's lymphomas EXCEPT

(A) exploratory celiotomy for staging
(B) splenectomy for localized splenic involvement
(C) resection of small intestinal lesions
(D) excisional lymph node biopsy
(E) total gastrectomy for lesions localized to the stomach

176. All the following statements about hepatic resectional management of metastatic colorectal cancers are true EXCEPT that

(A) a small, solitary metastasis recognized at the time of colectomy should be removed by local excision or wedge resection
(B) patients with solitary metastases are those most likely to be cured
(C) mortality of lobectomy for resection of metastatic foci is less than 10 percent
(D) patient survival after surgery for metachronous metastases is significantly higher than with surgery for synchronous metastases
(E) 5-year survival rates of 20 to 40 percent can be expected when resection is possible

177. In centers with experienced personnel, 1-year liver transplant survival is now approximately

(A) 95 percent
(B) 80 percent
(C) 65 percent
(D) 50 percent
(E) 35 percent

178. The subpopulations of T lymphocytes interact to effect the cellular immune response to tumor and allograft antigens by all the following mechanisms EXCEPT

(A) lymphokine release
(B) antigen recognition
(C) inhibition of B-cell development
(D) stimulation of B-cell differentiation
(E) IgG immunoglobulin production

179. Immunosuppression for transplantation has resulted in a higher incidence of all the following tumors EXCEPT

(A) cervical carcinoma
(B) basal cell carcinoma of the skin
(C) squamous cell carcinoma of the skin
(D) carcinoma of the colon
(E) B-cell lymphoma

180. The primary mechanism of action of cyclosporine A is inhibition of

(A) macrophage function
(B) antibody production
(C) interleukin 1 production
(D) interleukin 2 production
(E) cytotoxic T-cell effectiveness

181. The utility of adjuvant radiotherapy in the treatment of tumors is limited by all the following considerations EXCEPT

(A) injury to normal tissues
(B) oncogenic potential of treatment
(C) activation of T lymphocytes
(D) restriction to regional therapy
(E) systemic subclinical disease

182. An 11-year-old girl presents to your office because of a family history of medullary carcinoma of the thyroid. Physical examination is normal. You would perform all the following tests EXCEPT

(A) urine vanillylmandelic acid (VMA)
(B) serum calcitonin
(C) serum gastrin
(D) serum calcium
(E) pentagastrin stimulation

183. Proposed oncogene mechanisms include all the following EXCEPT

(A) production of mutant proteins that are important in the control of cell replication
(B) increase in the activity or density of cellular receptors for growth factors
(C) damage to DNA, thereby eliminating the transcription of a gene
(D) increase in the numbers of copies of the oncogene per cell, thereby increasing the gene product
(E) translocation of the gene to a new chromosomal environment, thereby changing its control and regulation

Questions 184–185

A 30-year-old primigravida complains of headaches, restlessness, sweating, and tachycardia. She is 8 months pregnant and her BP is 200/120.

184. Appropriate work-up might include all the following EXCEPT

(A) urine for epinephrine
(B) urine for norepinephrine
(C) chest x-ray
(D) abdominal CT scan
(E) abdominal ultrasonogram

185. Appropriate treatment might consist of all the following EXCEPT

(A) urgent excision of the tumor
(B) urgent excision of the tumor and a therapeutic abortion
(C) phenoxybenzamine and propranolol followed by a c-section and an elective excision of the tumor after delivery
(D) phenoxybenzamine and propranolol followed by a combined c-section and excision of the tumor
(E) metyrosine (Demser) blockade followed by a combined c-section and excision of the tumor

186. Which of the following statements concerning the human histocompatibility antigenic type (HLA) is true?

(A) Both class I and class II antigens can be detected serologically
(B) Donor-recipient identity at the A, B, and D loci precludes the need for immunosuppression
(C) It is used to induce chimerism in renal transplant recipients
(D) Tissue typing for HLA detects preformed cytotoxic antibodies to donor tissue
(E) HLA matching correlates with graft survival very well

Questions 187–191

A 27-year-old diabetic, hypertensive woman who has been receiving hemodialysis for 2 years is admitted to the hospital for cadaveric renal transplantation. She is blood type B and has had four transfusions of packed cells over the preceding 6 months.

187. Which of the following factors would preclude transplantation?

(A) Positive crossmatch
(B) Donor blood type O
(C) Two-antigen HLA match with donor
(D) Blood pressure of 180/100 mmHg
(E) Hemoglobin level of 8.2 g/100 ml

188. On the second postoperative day, the patient remains oliguric, but there is good perfusion on the renal scan and no hydronephrosis. The most commonly used immunosuppressive therapy at this time would be administration of

(A) cyclosporine A alone
(B) cyclosporine A and steroids
(C) cyclosporine A, steroids, and azathioprine
(D) OKT3 and steroids
(E) cyclophosphamide and steroids

189. On the 14th posttransplant day, the recipient's temperature rises to 38.5°C (101°F). The serum creatinine level, previously 1.0 mg/100 ml, is 1.6 mg/100 ml. Renal scan shows good perfusion with delayed excretion. Ultrasound reveals a mildly enlarged transplant kidney with a small fluid collection near the upper pole. The white blood cell count is $3800/mm^3$ and the platelet count is $65{,}000/mm^3$. Appropriate management at this time might include all the following EXCEPT

(A) increased administration of prednisone
(B) administration of azathioprine
(C) administration of antilymphocyte globulin (ALG)
(D) administration of OKT3
(E) percutaneous needle biopsy of the graft

190. On the 21st posttransplant day, the patient is being maintained on cyclosporine A, azathioprine, and prednisone. The serum creatinine level is 1.2 mg/100 ml, temperature is 38.5°C (101°F), and ultrasound shows a normal size kidney with a somewhat enlarged fluid collection at the upper pole. The renal scan is normal, white blood cell count is 13,500/mm^3, and platelet count is 160,000/mm^3. There is a hazy left lower lobe infiltrate on chest x-ray. The appropriate immediate therapeutic maneuvers would be

(A) withhold azathioprine, maintain cyclosporine, decrease prednisone dosage, aspirate the fluid collection, and perform bronchoscopy
(B) withhold azathioprine and cyclosporine, decrease prednisone dosage, and perform transplant nephrectomy with drainage of the fluid collection
(C) continue azathioprine and cyclosporine, decrease prednisone dosage, aspirate the fluid collection, and monitor serial antiviral antibody titers
(D) maintain immunosuppressive drugs, perform plasmapheresis with infusion of granulocytes, and begin antibiotics
(E) maintain immunosuppressive drugs, perform a bone marrow biopsy, and begin antibiotics

191. On the 40th postoperative day, the patient feels well but is somewhat hypertensive. She had been started on ketoconazole for oral candidiasis. The serum creatinine level is 2.0 mg/100 ml and the serum cyclosporine level is 275 ng/ml. There are no fluid collections found on ultrasound. Appropriate initial management at this time would be to

(A) perform an immediate biopsy with management dependent on frozen section results
(B) discontinue immunosuppression with a diagnosis of systemic candidal infection
(C) decrease the cyclosporine and increase the prednisone
(D) start OKT3
(E) administer a bolus with intravenous steroids and plan biopsy in 3 days if there is no improvement

Questions 192–193

A 54-year-old woman is admitted to the hospital because of mental changes and elevated calcium and alkaline phosphatase levels.

192. Initial work-up would include all the following EXCEPT

(A) complete blood count (CBC)
(B) mammogram
(C) parathormone (PTH) level
(D) dexamethasone suppression test
(E) bone scan

193. Therapy may include all the following EXCEPT

(A) hydration with normal saline
(B) furosemide (Lasix)
(C) cortisone
(D) potassium replacement
(E) digitalis

194. Prior to performing an open biopsy of an enlarged cervical lymph node, all the following tests should be done EXCEPT

(A) sinus x-ray
(B) CT scan of the head and neck
(C) bone marrow biopsy
(D) nasopharyngoscopy
(E) indirect laryngoscopy

195. Following intravenous administration of systemic chemotherapy,

(A) subcutaneous extravasation of carmustine (BCNU) or 5-fluorouracil (5-FU) usually causes ulceration
(B) doxorubicin extravasation rarely causes serious ulceration because the agent binds quickly to tissue nucleic acid
(C) serious and progressive ulceration can be expected following extravasation of vincristine or vinblastine
(D) problems of wound healing should be anticipated if systemic 5-FU therapy is begun less than 2 weeks postoperatively
(E) administration of folinic acid ''rescues'' patients from most of the toxicity of methotrexate, but has little beneficial effect on the impairment of wound healing

196. Immunotherapy of solid tumors in humans is

(A) effective in treatment of malignant melanoma
(B) dependent upon activation of the host's cellular immune system
(C) limited by toxicity to rapidly dividing normal host tissues
(D) dependent upon the presence of tumor-specific antigens
(E) currently clinically useful only for nonresectable cancers

197. Which of the following immunologic cells kills tumor cells in an immunologically specific manner?

(A) Macrophage
(B) Cytotoxic T lymphocyte
(C) Natural killer cell
(D) Polymorphonuclear leukocyte
(E) Helper T lymphocyte

198. Surgical treatment for ovarian carcinoma includes all the following EXCEPT

(A) bilateral salpingo-oophorectomy
(B) hysterectomy
(C) cytologic examination of ascites
(D) liver biopsy
(E) excision of peritoneal metastases

199. Preoperative radiation therapy increases the long-term survival rate for locally advanced malignancies of which of the following tissues?

(A) Larynx
(B) Lung
(C) Kidney
(D) Bone
(E) Rectum

Questions 200–201

A 24-year-old woman presents with lethargy, anorexia, tachypnea, and weakness. Laboratory studies reveal a BUN of 150 mg/100 ml, serum creatinine of 16 mg/100 ml, and a potassium of 6.2 mEq/L. Chest x-ray shows increased pulmonary vascularity and a dilated heart.

200. Management of this patient would include all the following EXCEPT

(A) peritoneal dialysis
(B) creation of a forearm arteriovenous fistula
(C) sodium polystyrene sulfonate (Kayexalate) enemas
(D) a 100-g protein diet
(E) renal biopsy

201. In the course of 3 months' treatment, the patient's congestive heart failure resolves, the lethargy and weakness diminish markedly, and she is able to return to work part-time. Family immune profile studies reveal that her mother and father each are haplotype identical with regard to HLA antigens and that her sister is a six antigen match. The patient at this time should be urged to

(A) continue hemodialysis three times a week
(B) undergo cadaveric renal transplantation
(C) accept a kidney transplant from her sister
(D) accept a kidney transplant from her father
(E) accept a kidney transplant from her mother

DIRECTIONS: Each question below contains four suggested responses of which **one or more** is correct. Select

A	if	**1, 2, and 3**	are correct
B	if	**1 and 3**	are correct
C	if	**2 and 4**	are correct
D	if	**4**	is correct
E	if	**1, 2, 3, and 4**	are correct

202. True statements about transmission of AIDS in a health-care setting and recommendations to reduce the risk of transmission include

(1) a freshly prepared solution of dilute chlorine bleach adequately decontaminates clothing
(2) all needles should be capped immediately after use
(3) endoscopes should be cleaned and gas sterilized after use on an HIV seropositive patient
(4) double gloving is highly recommended

203. Correct statements concerning the effects of radiation include which of the following?

(1) The excess risk of radiogenic cancer from diagnostic radiologic studies is estimated to be one case per million procedures per year
(2) Cellular hypoxia increases sensitivity to radiation
(3) The condition of the cell nucleus in relation to its mitotic cycle determines cell sensitivity to radiation
(4) In addition to natural background radiation, the safe limit for an average person is 0.5 rad per year (15 r/30 yr)

204. Correct statements concerning the behavior of tumor cells include which of the following?

(1) About 25 percent of the tumor cells invading the central circulation remain viable beyond 24 hours
(2) It takes 1 billion cells for a tumor to become clinically detectable (1 cc)
(3) Most cells cloned from the same tumors have similar metastatic potential
(4) Local invasion is related to lytic enzymes produced by the tumor cells

205. Monoclonal antibodies produced by hybridomas are useful for

(1) determination of T-lymphocyte subpopulations
(2) screening blood for tumor associated antigens
(3) reversal of renal allograft rejection
(4) targeting toxins to tumors

206. Characterization of T- and B-cell subpopulations by monoclonal antibodies is important for diagnosing

(1) acquired immune deficiency syndrome (AIDS)
(2) non-Hodgkin's lymphoma
(3) leukemia
(4) Hodgkin's lymphoma

207. Regarding cancer therapy with interleukin 2 (IL2) and lymphokine-activated killer (LAK) cells,

(1) there is a marked increase in the peripheral lymphocyte count
(2) response rates of greater than 20 percent have been shown in melanoma, renal cell carcinoma, and non-Hodgkin's lymphoma
(3) examination of responsive tumors after such treatment shows infiltration of large, activated T cells
(4) LAK cell infusion without in vivo IL2 is nearly as effective as the combination

208. Cardiac transplants differ from renal transplants in that

(1) negative lymphocyte crossmatch is not necessary in heart transplantation
(2) cadaveric graft survival is significantly lower with heart transplants
(3) cadaveric kidneys can be preserved for substantially longer periods than hearts
(4) simple hypothermic preservation is inadequate for kidneys but satisfactory for hearts

SUMMARY OF DIRECTIONS

A	B	C	D	E
1,2,3 only	1,3 only	2,4 only	4 only	All are correct

209. True statements concerning the process involving the rejecting kidney shown below include that

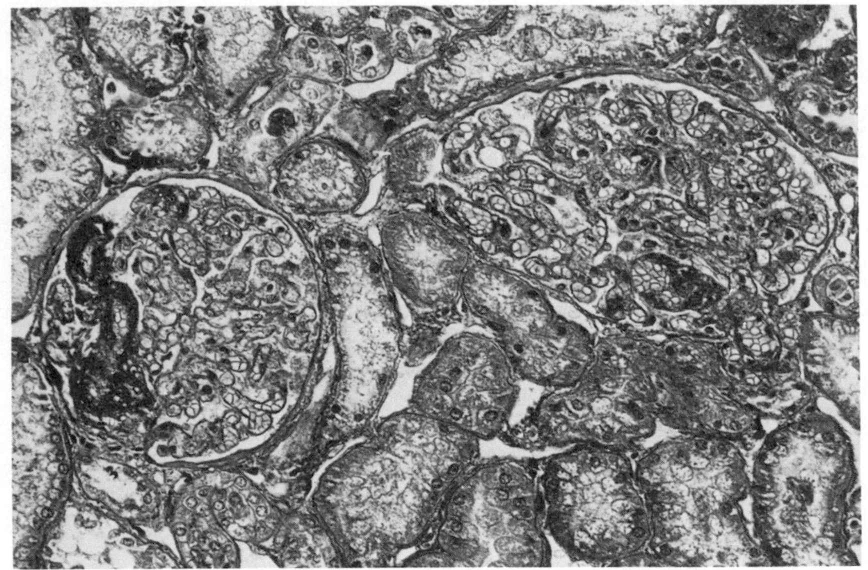

(1) it is mediated by antibodies against donor HLA antigens
(2) it can be avoided by performing cytotoxicity testing by incubating the recipient's serum with the donor lymphocytes
(3) it is manifest grossly by a swollen, pale kidney at the time of transplant surgery
(4) this form of rejection is associated with disseminated intravascular coagulation (DIC)

210. Contraindications to liver transplantation include

(1) pneumonia
(2) acute hepatitis B
(3) extrahepatic malignancy
(4) alcoholic cirrhosis

211. Testicular carcinomas requiring retroperitoneal lymph node dissection include

(1) embryonal carcinoma
(2) seminoma
(3) teratocarcinoma
(4) choriocarcinoma

212. Correct statements concerning human bone marrow transplants include which of the following?

(1) Marrow is highly immunogenic and easily rejected by the nonimmunosuppressed host
(2) Experimental techniques have shown promise for the induction of tolerance to organ allografts
(3) The major impediment to successful marrow grafting is the graft-versus-host response
(4) Marrow transplant must be performed with low level immunosuppression to enhance the degree of chimerism

213. Correct statements concerning cancer and nutrition include which of the following?

(1) Levels of nitrates in food and drinking water are positively correlated with the incidence of gastric cancer
(2) Regular ingestion of vitamin C from childhood probably inhibits formation of gastric carcinogens
(3) Consumption of excessive amounts of animal dietary fats is associated with increased incidences of pancreatic, breast, and prostatic cancers
(4) Nutritional support of cancer patients improves response of the tumor to chemotherapy

214. Five-year survival rates in excess of 20 percent may be expected following resection of pulmonary metastases if

(1) no other organ metastases are present
(2) lung lesions are solitary
(3) the patient's condition and tumor location are favorable
(4) the tumor doubling time is less than 20 days

DIRECTIONS: The group of questions below consists of four lettered headings followed by a set of numbered items. For each numbered item select

A	if the item is associated with	(A) **only**
B	if the item is associated with	(B) **only**
C	if the item is associated with	**both** (A) and (B)
D	if the item is associated with	**neither** (A) nor (B)

Each lettered heading may be used **once, more than once, or not at all.**

Questions 215–219

(A) Fluid from which human immunodeficiency virus (HIV) has been isolated
(B) Fluid implicated in the transmission of HIV
(C) Both
(D) Neither

215. Blood

216. Urine

217. Semen

218. Vaginal secretions

219. Sweat

DIRECTIONS: The group of questions below consists of lettered headings followed by a set of numbered items. For each numbered item select the **one** lettered heading with which it is **most** closely associated. Each lettered heading may be used **once, more than once, or not at all.**

Questions 220–224

All the immunosuppressants currently used to prevent or treat allograft rejection have significant deleterious side effects. For each of the complications below, match the agent.

(A) Azathioprine
(B) Corticosteroids
(C) Antilymphocyte serum
(D) Cyclophosphamide
(E) Cyclosporine

220. Nephrotoxicity

221. Hepatotoxicity

222. Testicular atrophy

223. Anaphylactoid reaction

224. Gastrointestinal ulceration

Transplants, Immunology, and Oncology

Answers

173. The answer is C. *(Schwartz, ed 5. pp 342–343.)* In vitro immunologic techniques provide a sensitive tool for the assay of tumor-associated antigens. The ultimate goals of this methodology are early detection and tumor cell specific immunotherapy. Cellular immunity can be demonstrated by the ability of lymphocytes to kill tumor cells (lymphocyte-mediated cytotoxicity), tumor antigen stimulation of lymphocyte blastogenesis, inhibition of macrophage migration by tumor antigens, and delayed cutaneous hypersensitivity reactions to tumor antigens. Immunodiffusion techniques have been useful in identifying antibodies to tumor-associated antigens.

174. The answer is C. *(Schwartz, ed 5. p 332.)* There has been a steady increase in the death rate from lung cancer in this country since 1930. The rate has gone from 18 to 67 per 100,000 in men and from 4.6 to 16.6 per 100,000 in women. Over that time span, there has been a drastic decrease in the death rate from stomach and uterine cancer; this decrease has been attributed to improved surveillance and therapy. There has been a mild increase in both the incidence and mortality of pancreatic cancer. Breast cancer and colon cancer death rates have been stable over the last 40 years.

175. The answer is E. *(Copeland, pp 640–641, 644–646.)* Although somewhat controversial, staging laparotomy is generally recommended for many patients with non-Hodgkin's lymphoma whose disease is localized to a single lymph node region. Since, however, most patients with non-Hodgkin's lymphoma (over 90 percent) have anatomically disseminated disease at time of presentation, this issue is not often germane. Treatment usually consists of combination chemotherapy and radiation, but surgery is important in establishing the diagnosis and in resection of extranodal lymphomas. These may arise in the gastrointestinal tract, bone, soft tissue, skin, and nasopharynx. Lymphomas constitute 3 percent of all malignant gastric tumors. Ninety percent of these lymphomas are non-Hodgkin's. For early lesions, resections can achieve a 30 percent 5-year survival rate. If a total gastrectomy is necessary to remove the lesion, resection should not be performed and chemoradiotherapy should be employed.

176. The answer is D. *(Copeland, pp 618–620.)* Ten percent of patients with colorectal cancer have liver metastases at time of initial presentation. Thirty to forty percent of patients with recurrent disease have liver metastases. Patients with metastatic disease localized to resectable portions of the liver who are suitable candidates for surgery should undergo appropriate local excision or lobectomy since 5-year survival rates of 20 to 40 percent can be anticipated. Patients with solitary metastases have the most favorable prognosis, but cures after lobectomy for multiple metastases are also reported. Operative mortality of less than 10 percent should be expected after lobectomy and less than 5 percent for local or wedge resections. Data from the Liver Tumor Study on colorectal hepatic metastases have shown no survival benefit to patients with synchronous as opposed to metachronous disease.

177. The answer is B. *(Schwartz, ed 5. p 426.)* With the introduction of cyclosporine in the early 1980s and the rapidly accumulated experience with liver transplantation, graft and patient survivals have improved markedly. In the azathioprine and steroid era, 1-year graft survival was in the range of 25 percent. More recently, most centers are experiencing 1-year graft survival rates of approximately 80 percent.

178. The answer is E. *(Schwartz, ed 5. pp 393–396.)* T lymphocytes include a number of subpopulations that interact with each other as well as with B cells in effecting the host immune responses to foreign antigens, including those present in tumor and allograft tissues. T cells do not produce antibodies, although they do assist in B-cell function by producing B-cell–directed lymphokines in response to specific antigen, thereby stimulating B stem cells to differentiate into antibody-producing cells (T helper functions). Another T-cell subgroup, the suppressor cell, inhibits both the development of B cells and the generation of T effector cells. T effector cells are responsible for the cytotoxic function central to graft rejection and destruction of tumor cells. Lymphokines, released by various T-cell subpopulations, affect the function of white cells, including macrophages, polymorphonuclear leukocytes, and other T cells.

179. The answer is D. *(Schwartz, ed 5. pp 409–412.)* Most of the spontaneous cancers found in immunosuppressed transplant patients are either epithelial or lymphoid in origin. Of the epithelial tumors the most common are those of the cervix, lip, and skin (both basal and squamous). The incidence of cervical cancer is four times higher than in the general population; that of skin cancer forty times higher. Whether this is a consequence of herpes virus transformation is unknown. B-cell lymphoma is 350 times more common in this immunosuppressed population. It is a highly malignant form of lymphoma and affects the CNS in 50 percent of cases.

180. The answer is D. *(Schwartz, ed 5. p 406.)* Cyclosporine is a highly effective immunosuppressive agent produced by fungi. It is more specific than the anti-inflammatory agents such as steroids or the antiproliferative agents such as azathioprine. The eftectiveness of cyclosporine in preventing allograft rejection is related to its ability to inhibit interleukin 2 production. Without interleukin 2 from helper T cells, there is no clonal expansion of alloantigen-directed cytotoxic T cells and no stimulation of antibody production by B cells.

181. The answer is C. *(Schwartz, ed 5. pp 362–365.)* The use of adjuvant radiotherapy in the treatment of tumors is restricted by its toxicity to bone marrow and other normal tissues, such as the lung and intestinal tract. Treatment must, therefore, be limited both in terms of dosage and region to be irradiated. Since total body irradiation is generally not feasible, subclinical tumor implants that lie in tissues outside the irradiated field will escape therapy. The oncogenic effects of irradiation are well known and constitute a lifelong risk for those patients with a potential for extended survival. T cells are radiosensitive; therapy can effect a prolonged T-cell depletion that may interfere with the host immune defenses against tumor growth and spread.

182. The answer is C. *(Schwartz, ed 5. pp 1636–1638.)* Medullary carcinomas occur in families as part of syndromes called multiple endocrine neoplasia (MEN), type IIA and type IIB. MEN-IIA consists of multicentric medullary thyroid cancer, pheochromocytomas or adrenal medullary hyperplasia, and hyperparathyroidism. MEN-IIB consists of medullary cancer, pheochromocytoma and mucosal neuromas, gangliomas, and a Marfan-like habitus. These patients may develop medullary carcinoma at a very young age, and any patient with MEN-IIB should be assumed to have medullary cancer until proven otherwise. Patients are followed carefully for pheochromocytoma with urine VMA, for hyperparathyroidism with serum calcium, and for medullary carcinoma with serum calcitonin. However, as some patients have a normal basal calcitonin, a pentagastrin or calcium infusion test should be performed in these high-risk patients. Gastrin levels should be obtained in patients thought to have MEN-I syndrome (pituitary, parathyroid, and pancreatic tumors) or Zollinger-Ellison syndrome.

183. The answer is C. *(Schwartz, ed 5. pp 336–338.)* There are several known oncogenes that have been circumstantially linked to human cancers. These genes have been conserved across great evolutionary distances. The known mechanisms of oncogene action are active processes rather than elimination of a gene product. The *ras* gene undergoes mutation in two known hot spots. These point mutations produce a membrane protein that functions inappropriately in the control of cell growth. The oncogene family that includes the *src* gene codes for proteins that have tyrosine kinase activity. Decreases in tyrosine kinase activity markedly influence surface receptor response to growth factors such as platelet-derived growth factor, epidermal growth factor, and insulinlike growth factor. The N-*myc* oncogene demonstrates the principle of amplification. The overall prognosis in neuroblastoma correlates with the number of N-*myc* copies per cell. The more repetitive copies of N-*myc* there are per cell, the worse the prognosis becomes. Chromosomal abnormalities in Burkitt's lymphoma and chronic myelogenous leukemia (Philadelphia chromosome) demonstrate translocation. In Burkitt's lymphoma, the long arm of chromosome 8, which contains the C-*myc* oncogene, is translocated to chromosome 14. This results in abnormal regulation of the expression of C-*myc*.

184–185. The answers are: 184-D, 185-B. *(Schwartz, ed 5. pp 1588–1595.)* This young pregnant woman presents with the symptoms of a pheochromocytoma. These tumors can become initially symptomatic during pregnancy. A noninvasive workup should be performed. Ultrasonography of the abdomen is frequently sufficient to localize the tumor to the right or left adrenal; an abdominal CT scan with its large dose of radiation should be avoided in pregnancy. The treatment can be early excision of the pheochromocytoma, and in three cases in pregnant women this was done with survival of two of the three infants. A therapeutic abortion, especially at 8 months, is not indicated. The more current approach is α- and β-adrenergic blockade followed by vaginal delivery or c-section with excision of the tumor at the same time as delivery or electively after delivery. Metyrosine (Demser) inhibits tyrosine hydroxylase and results in a decrease in endogenous levels of catecholamines. This form of treatment is also acceptable.

186. The answer is A. *(Schwartz, ed 5. pp 388–391.)* The major histocompatibility complex (MHC) is located on chromosome 6 in humans. Human leukocyte antigens (HLA) are the protein products of this chromosome region. Antigens that trigger the proliferation of allogeneic lymphocytes, called class II antigens, are expressions of the HLA-D locus; antigens that cannot trigger this lymphocytic proliferation, class I antigens, are expressions of the HLA-A and -B loci. Both antigen classes are detectable serologically. Because there are genes on other chromosomes outside the MHC that code for weaker histocompatibility loci, identity at HLA-A, -B, and -D, even in living related donor-recipient pairs, does not mean rejection will not occur. Immunosuppression is still necessary. Only identical twins are truly perfect matches. With the improvement of immunosuppressive techniques heralded by cyclosporine, the beneficial effects of tissue typing are not as evident as in the past. When all six of the antigens tested for are matched, there is a demonstrable improvement in graft survival. Preformed cytotoxic antibodies are not detected by HLA typing and must be assayed by the lymphocyte crossmatch test prior to transplantation to avoid acute humoral rejection. Chimerism develops when donor and recipient strain marrow cells coexist in a single host and is not induced by transfer of HLA protein.

187–191. The answers are: 187-A, 188-D, 189-B, 190-A, 191-C. *(Schwartz, ed 5. pp 403–412, 440–452.)* A positive crossmatch means that the recipient has circulating antibodies that are cytotoxic to donor strain lymphocytes. This incompatibility, which almost always leads to an acute humoral rejection of the graft, precludes transplantation. Blood type matching prior to organ allograft is similar to crossmatching prior to transfusion; O is the universal donor and AB the universal recipient. Minor blood group factors do not appear to act as histocompatibility antigens. Matching of HLA antigens in cadaveric renal transplants may improve graft survival, but the impact is relatively minor. While attempts are made to pair recipient and donor by tissue typing, a two antigen match is perfectly acceptable and even zero antigen matches can be transplanted with good results. Neither hypertension nor anemia is a contraindication to transplantation; indeed, hypertension may be cured or ameliorated following successful transplantation. Patients with end-stage renal failure generally are anemic and can be transfused, if necessary, intra- or postoperatively. Anemia generally also improves following transplantation because of increased erythropoietin production by the graft.

The differential diagnosis of the oliguric patient in the early posttransplant period includes technical error with the vascular or ureteral anastomosis, accelerated rejection, or acute tubular necrosis (ATN). Good perfusion on the renal scan eliminates the arterial anastomosis as the problem and makes antibody-mediated rejection very unlikely. The lack of hydronephrosis eliminates ureteral obstruction as the source of oliguria. ATN is the diagnosis by exclusion. Most transplant centers will
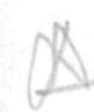
withhold cyclosporine in the setting of ATN because of the known potentiation of cyclosporine nephrotoxicity in this setting. Although some transplant centers will treat with azathioprine and steroids in this setting, most are now using an antilymphocyte preparation such as OKT3 or ALG until the ATN resolves. At that time, cyclosporine therapy is initiated.

The findings on the 14th day suggest that the patient has suffered a rejection episode. Because of the depressed white blood cell and platelet counts, azathioprine must be withheld to avoid further bone marrow suppression. Rejection treatment in this setting generally includes increased steroid administration. Definitive diagnosis by biopsy is indicated, inasmuch as infection and rejection can be confused or may coexist. With infection present, immunosuppressants must be withheld or decreased, regardless of the effect on the graft survival. If rejection is confirmed by biopsy and there is no response to steroids, then an antilymphocyte preparation is usually started. ALG and OKT3 are both very effective agents. ALG will frequently cause thrombocytopenia and therefore OKT3 is currently being used more often.

Temperature elevation, chest film findings, and lack of evidence for rejection suggest the presence of pneumonitis. The first priority is the patient's survival, not allograft salvage. The current mortality level in transplant patients is approximately 5 to 10 percent, with infection the major cause of death. Immunosuppressed patients are at high risk for viral, fungal, and protozoal infections, all of which are difficult to diagnose. Aggressive measures, including bronchoscopy, aspiration, and biopsy, are imperative for appropriate diagnosis and treatment. Immunosuppressant dosages must be reduced. Cyclosporine is the most specific of the agents this patient is being treated with. It decreases antibacterial defense mechanisms less than do steroids or azathioprine and can sometimes be maintained throughout the course of a controlled infection. Percutaneous drainage of perirenal fluid collections for culture may reveal an infected lymphocele as a coexisting or primary infectious locus. Transplant nephrectomy is not necessary at this stage since the graft may survive the period of infection despite withdrawal of immunosuppressants.

Cyclosporine nephrotoxicity must be suspected whenever there is an asymptomatic rise in serum creatinine. Many drugs, one of which is ketoconazole, influence the hepatic metabolism of cyclosporine and can produce elevated serum levels (therapeutic range is 100 to 200 ng/ml) without dosage changes. In the setting described on the 40th postoperative day, the cyclosporine dose should be decreased. Many transplant surgeons would simultaneously increase other immunosuppressive agents to guard against rejection. If there is no improvement in serum creatinine after this step, then renal biopsy is indicated.

192–193. The answers are: 192-D, 193-E. *(Schwartz, ed 5. pp 352, 1645–1660.)* Mental changes and hypercalcemia may be the presenting symptoms of either hyperparathyroidism or cancer. The tumors most often associated with hypercalcemia are those of the lung, breast, kidney, and uterus and some sarcomas and hemopoietic neoplasms, especially multiple myeloma. Therefore, the work-up would consist of a CBC, chest x-ray, mammogram, bone scan, PTH levels, and possibly more directed examinations such as an intravenous pyelogram (IVP) and CT scan. A PTH level would be elevated in parathyroid disease, but low in metastatic carcinoma. A dexamethasone suppression test is used to assess the production of cortisol by an adrenal cortical adenoma or carcinoma.

The therapy of hypercalcemia is based on increasing calcium excretion and limiting calcium intake. Since calcium excretion parallels that of sodium, it is important to rehydrate all patients with normal saline. This can be done at a rapid rate (200 ml/hr) providing renal and cardiac status is good. Lasix is used to help calcium and fluid excretion. Cortisone is especially useful in the treatment of myeloma and various leukemias and lymphomas, but it takes 7 to 10 days to work. Most hypercalcemic patients are also hypokalemic and will require potassium replacement especially when hydration and Lasix are begun. Calcium and digitalis are synergistic on the myocardium and conducting system. The drug should be stopped and restarted in small doses after checking calcium levels and ECGs.

194. The answer is C. *(Schwartz, ed 5. pp 354–355, 584, 612–613.)* Isolated enlarged cervical lymph nodes present a diagnostic problem. They may be involved with neoplasms that originate in the hypopharynx, piriform sinus, larynx, or thyroid or they may contain a lymphoma. It is important to ascertain the location of the primary neoplasm prior to excision, because curative surgery may involve a radical neck dissection, which would be complicated by a previous biopsy. There is also fear of tumor spread in an open biopsy. Bone marrow biopsy is not indicated prior to lymph node biopsy. It is done as part of the staging procedure, after a diagnosis of lymphoma has been made. Needle aspiration cytology is now being used more widely. It can often diagnose carcinomas, but is rarely useful for the diagnosis of lymphoma.

195. The answer is D. *(Falcone, Surg Clin North Am 64:779–794, 1984. Rudolph, J Clin Oncol 5:1116–1126, 1987.)* Since chemotherapy is generally most effective in killing rapidly dividing cells, the rapidly dividing cells of a fresh surgical wound should be in jeopardy when chemotherapy is given in the early postoperative period. Each of the phases of normal wound healing are theoretically at risk from one or another class of chemotherapeutic agents. Immediately following wounding, inflammation and vascular permeability lead to fibrin deposition and polymorphonuclear neutrophil (PMN), monocyte, and platelet influx. Macrophages are attracted by the activated complement system. By the fourth day, the proliferative phase begins and for the next 20 days fibroblasts produce mucopolysaccharides and collagen. Cross-linking of the collagen fibers then continues for several months in the maturation phase. It seems logical to delay antineoplastic agents for 10 to 14 days unless there are compelling clinical indications (e.g., superior vena cava syndrome) for more urgent treatment. Administration of folinic acid simultaneously with methotrexate normalizes wound healing. Extravasation of chemotherapeutic agents during intravenous administration may result in severe ulceration and sloughing. The nature of the injury is largely related to the nucleic acid–binding characteristics of the agent. Those agents that do not bind to tissue nucleic acid (vincristine, vinblastine, nitrogen mustard, BCNU, 5-FU) generally cause only local damage resulting from the immediate injury. These substances are quickly metabolized or inactivated, and usually patterns of wound healing can be expected. On the other hand, agents that bind the nucleic acid (doxorubicin, dactinomycin, mitomycin C, mithramycin, and daunorubicin) cause not only immediate toxic reaction in the tissues but, unless excised, continuing and progressive tissue damage. Though some authors have reported success with elevation and ice packs, most recommend surgical excision if there is severe pain, any sign of early necrosis, or significant blistering.

196. The answer is D. *(Schwartz, ed 5. pp 373–378.)* In theory, immunotherapy provides the best available approach to cancer treatment. Provided a tumor specific antigen is present to distinguish the neoplastic cell from normal tissue, it should be possible to develop cytotoxic antibodies or cells to destroy, selectively, only those cells bearing the tumor antigen. This approach would circumvent the toxicity of chemo- and radiotherapeutic treatment modalities to rapidly dividing normal host tissues such as bone marrow and intestinal mucosa. The methods tested to date include active immunotherapy through injection of inactivated tumor cells, passive immunotherapy conferred by injection of cells and sera from sensitized secondary hosts, and nonspecific enhancement of the tumor host's own immune surveillance system by methods such as BCG treatment. To date, however, none of these approaches has proved clinically effective.

197. The answer is B. *(Schwartz, ed 5. pp 342–343.)* Unlike the granulocyte line, T lymphocytes express the T-cell receptor. This receptor imports antigen specificity to T cells. The T-helper cell, when stimulated by interleukin 1 and antigens, produces various lymphokines that ultimately produce effector cells. One of these effector cells is the cytotoxic T cell, which will kill cells expressing specific antigens including viral tumor and nonbiological antigens. Macrophages and natural killer cells have some tumoricidal activity; however, this is not specific for tumors.

198. The answer is D. *(Schwartz, ed 5. pp 1817–1821.)* Reduction of tumor mass in ovarian carcinoma is helpful in improving the response to chemotherapy and radiation. The primary therapy consists of hysterectomy and bilateral salpingo-oophorectomy. If ascites is present it should be examined for malignant cells. All local peritoneal implants should be removed. However, pelvic exenteration, with removal of the bladder and rectum, has generally not improved survival. Liver biopsy is not indicated. If localized liver metastases are present, a limited liver resection may be performed.

199. The answer is A. *(Schwartz, ed 5. pp 366, 601–603.)* Preoperative irradiation has been useful in treating certain tumors, either to increase the cure rate or decrease the incidence of local recurrence. For laryngeal malignancies confined to the true vocal cords, radiotherapy alone may result in 5-year survivals of over 90 percent. With local invasion, laryngectomy and radical neck dissection are the preferred management, but pretreatment with radiotherapy may increase the cure rate. Preoperative radiotherapy of rectal cancers, which may convert inoperable to operable tumors and decrease local recurrence rates, has not been shown to increase long-term survival rates. Preoperative radiotherapy for tumors of bone, kidney, and lung has had no demonstrable beneficial effect.

200–201. The answers are: 200-D, 201-C. *(Schwartz, ed 5. pp 388–391, 440–443.)* Hemodialysis, rather than management by dietary manipulation alone, should be instituted in patients with end-stage renal failure whose serum creatinine is over 15 mg/100 ml or whose creatinine clearance is less than 3 ml/min. It is important that hemodialysis be initiated prior to the onset of uremic complications. These complications include hyperkalemia, congestive heart failure, peripheral neuropathy, severe hypertension, pericarditis, bleeding, and severe anemia. The uremic hyperkalemic patient in congestive heart failure may require emergency dialysis in addition to the standard conservative measures, which include (1) limitation of protein intake to less than 60 g/day and restriction of fluid intake; and (2) reduction of elevated serum potassium levels by insulin-glucose or sodium polystyrene sulfonate (Kayexalate) enema treatment. Arteriovenous fistulas require about 2 weeks to develop adequate size and flow. While awaiting maturation, temporary dialysis can be satisfactorily performed using either an external arteriovenous shunt or the peritoneal cavity. Renal biopsy would be performed in an attempt to obtain a diagnosis of the underlying renal disease.

Patients who are acceptable candidates for kidney transplantation usually should undergo this form of treatment rather than chronic hemodialysis, the mortality for which is now higher than for transplantation. Despite adequate dialysis, problems of neuropathy, bone disease, anemia, and hypertension remain difficult to manage. Compared with chronic dialysis, transplantation restores more patients to happier and more productive lives. It had been conjectured that, all other issues being equal, sex matching was important in the graft survival and that a mother-daughter graft was preferred to a father-daughter. Review of the current data does not support such a conclusion. The best graft survival rates for living related transplants—over 90 percent at 5 years—are obtained when all six histocompatibility loci are identical. All family members of potential transplant recipients should be tissue typed and the donor selected on the basis of closest match, if psychological and medical evaluation makes this feasible. With the development of cyclosporine-based immunosuppression, cadaveric kidney graft survival has approached that of living-related transplantation. There are some transplanters who believe that the slight improvement with living-related kidneys does not justify the risk to the donor and that these transplantations should no longer be performed.

202. The answer is B (1, 3). *(Telford, Surg Rounds 10:30–37, 1987.)* The risk of contracting AIDS is much less than the risk of contracting hepatitis B from a patient. Although the risk of transmission of AIDS in the health care setting is very low, there are reported cases of seroconversion after parenteral exposure. Particular precautions should be taken in operating upon patients who are known to be seropositive for HIV or who have known risk factors. Recommendations include elimination of inexperienced personnel or personnel with open lesions on body surfaces from the operating room. Disposable gowns, drapes, masks, and eye shields should be used. Clothing should be soaked in a dilute solution (1:10) of chlorine bleach prior to washing and personnel should shower after the procedure. Double gloving does not reduce the major intraoperative risk of needle puncture, which is the primary source of risk to the operating team. Needles should never be capped; an uncapped needle is less dangerous than are the maneuvers to recap needles.

203. The answer is B (1, 3). *(Hall, Cancer 55:2051–2057, 1985. Kohn, N Engl J Med 310:504–511, 1984.)* Among the basic principles of radiation biology are the observations that the sensitivity of mammalian cells to radiation varies with their position in the cell-division (mitotic) cycle. The percentage of cells killed by a given dose of x-rays or gamma rays is greatly increased by molecular oxygen; cells deficient in oxygen are resistant to radiation. Only about 30 percent of the biological damage from x-rays is due to the direct effects on the target molecule. The remainder is due to an indirect action mediated by free radicals and can be modified by free radical scavengers such as sulfhydryl. Workers at the Oak Ridge National Laboratory have identified the safe radiation limit for an average person as 0.17 rad per year, with a 30-year maximum of 5 rad. This is superimposed on the 12 rad the average

U.S. citizen will accumulate from natural sources by age 65. It is difficult to estimate cancer risk from radiation up to 10 rad above background since there is variation in risk per rad depending on dose, dose-rates, and the linear energy transfer (LET) of the radiation source. Low-LET radiation (i.e., gamma rays, x-rays, and beta rays) becomes less damaging to tissue per rad as the dose falls; high-LET radiation (e.g., neutrons and alpha particles) does not. The exposures from radiologic examinations are low-LET exposures in low-dose, low-dose-rate ranges and the risk associated with them is difficult to estimate. That risk has been estimated to be about one case of radiogenic cancer per million procedures per year.

204. The answer is C (2, 4). *(Fidler, Cancer Bull 39:126–131, 1987.)* Tumor metastases occur as a result of a complex process of tumor cell factors and host responses. At the lower limit of clinical detectability (1 cc), there are already 1 billion aggregated tumor cells. Experimental work confirms that cells or cell aggregates cultured from metastases are both biologically and immunologically heterogeneous, despite their similar histological appearance; they also have markedly variable potential for establishing viable metastases. In experimental models, 99 percent of radiolabeled tumor cells introduced into the circulation are dead by the end of the first 24 hours and less than 0.1 percent survive to produce metastases. Most injected tumor cells are destroyed by the mechanical stress of blood turbulence. Local invasion seems to be the consequence of several interrelated factors: the forcing of cords of cells along lower resistance paths as a result of mechanical pressure from the proliferating tumor mass; tumor cell motility; and, more clearly, specific tissue destruction and destabilization caused by destructive lytic enzymes produced by the neoplastic cells.

205. The answer is E (all). *(Schwartz, ed 5. pp 347, 406–408.)* Monoclonal antibodies are produced from the fusion of a mouse plasma cell and an "immortal" human myeloma cell. After the mouse has been immunized with a desired antigen, its spleen is removed and the plasma cells isolated. The fusion of these plasma cells with a myeloma cell results in a hybridoma that produces a clonal antibody. Monoclonal antibodies have been made to subpopulations of lymphocytes such as T-helper and T-suppressor cells. This advance has helped in understanding cell-to-cell interactions involved in rejection, hypersensitivity reactions, and immunosuppression. Antibodies to human lymphocytes (OKT3 + OKT4) have also been used therapeutically to treat rejection because they are felt to be more specific than antilymphocyte globulin (ALG). Monoclonal antibodies to human cancers have been used to screen for shed tumor antigens in patients with colon, ovarian, and breast cancers. They are also used to target toxins to tumors, thereby causing tumor necrosis with minimal side effects.

206. The answer is E (all). *(Schwartz, ed 5. p 347.)* Acquired immune deficiency syndrome (AIDS) is characterized by a reversal in the normal T-lymphocyte helper-to-suppressor ratio. Monoclonal antibodies are helpful in detecting this reversal in peripheral blood samples and in lymph node biopsies, especially when lymphocyte numbers and lymph node architecture appear normal. They are also important in the diagnosis of lymphomas, both non-Hodgkin's and Hodgkin's, and of leukemias. Monoclonal antibodies have been made to "TdT," a marker on immature B and T lymphocytes. This is especially helpful in differentiating lymphocytes from myelocytes in bone marrow biopsies, which is necessary in distinguishing acute myelocytic leukemia (AML) from acute lymphocytic leukemia (ALL). Monoclonal antibodies are also used for checking the clonal nature of B cells. If this is present, a lymphoma can be diagnosed even in the presence of a node that appears normal. A Hodgkin's lymphoma can be differentiated from a high-grade T lymphoma by the polyclonal nature of the cells in the former. Monoclonal antibodies to Reed-Sternberg cells have been made and are being used experimentally.

207. The answer is A (1, 2, 3). *(Lotze, Cancer 38:68–94, 1988.)* With the availability of recombinant IL2, multiple trials of cancer therapy with this lymphokine have been undertaken. The most successful trials include the reinfusion of in vivo IL2. Rosenberg's group has documented complete or partial responses in 33, 23, and 100 percent of renal cell, melanoma, and non-Hodgkin's lymphoma patients, respectively. Infusion of either LAK cells or IL2 alone was not nearly as effective. The therapy is not innocuous: there were 4 deaths among 106 patients treated. All patients exhibit a marked lymphocytosis, eosinophilia, fluid retention, fever, and decrease in peripheral vascular resistance.

208. The answer is B (1, 3). *(Schwartz, ed 5. pp 426–435.)* Cardiac transplantation has become an acceptable clinical treatment modality for selected patients with end-stage cardiac failure. Allograft survivals are now comparable to those of cadaveric renal transplants—approximately 70 percent at 1 year and 50 percent at 5 years as reported by the Stanford group. Although kidneys can be safely preserved by either hypothermic storage or hypothermic perfusion for periods up to 48 hours, donor hearts, protected by simple hypothermia, should be transplanted within 4 hours. For this reason the usual tissue-typing procedures utilized in kidney transplantation are impractical in cardiac transplantation. The role of prospective tissue-typing is not clear in cardiac transplantation and it is frequently not performed. In pairing donor and recipient for heart transplants there must be at least ABO blood group compatibility. Cyclosporine has improved results in both cardiac and renal transplantation despite its major drawback of dose-related nephrotoxicity.

209. The answer is E (all). *(Schwartz, ed 5. pp 398–403, 449–450.)* Hyperacute rejection is mediated by cytotoxic antibodies with subsequent triggering of the complement, coagulation, and kinin systems. It can occur during surgery after the clamps are released from the vascular anastomosis and the recipient's antibodies are exposed to the donor's passenger lymphocytes and kidney tissue. It is the cause of immediate and early oliguria and biopsies should be performed intraoperatively or early postoperatively. Hyperacute rejection is characterized pathologically by fibrin and platelet thrombosis and necrosis of the glomerular tufts, renal arterioles, and small arteries. Massive polymorphonuclear infiltrate with tubular necrosis occurs 24 to 36 hours after transplantation. The intravascular coagulation can rarely result in a systemic coagulopathy. Careful cross-matching can test for cytotoxic antibodies.

210. The answer is B (1, 3). *(Schwartz, ed 5. pp 421–442.)* The indications for liver transplantation have expanded in recent years with improvement in the results. The most common indication in adults is now chronic active hepatitis, followed by alcoholic and biliary cirrhosis. Other indications include acute fulminant hepatitis B, the Budd-Chiari syndrome, and genetic errors of metabolism. The most common indication in children is biliary atresia; these children frequently have had prior Kasai procedures. Transplantation for primary hepatic malignancies have been performed; the results, however, are poor. Contraindications include other malignancies or uncontrolled infections. Patients with alcoholic cirrhosis should be abstinent for 2 years or more.

211. The answer is B (1, 3). *(Schwartz, ed 5. pp 1768–1770.)* After radical orchiectomy, lymph node dissection is indicated in embryonal carcinoma, teratocarcinoma, and adult teratoma if there is no supradiaphragmatic spread. This dissection increases the 5-year survival and helps in staging. Seminoma is extremely radiosensitive and lymph node dissection is unnecessary. Choriocarcinoma is associated with pulmonary metastases in 81 percent of cases and is treated with chemotherapy.

212. The answer is A (1, 2, 3). *(Schwartz, ed 5. pp 417–418.)* Bone marrow cells are highly immunogenic. Successful engraftment requires the use of immunosuppressants that permit the transplanted cells not only to survive but also to mount a graft-versus-host response against recipient tissues. The graft-versus-host response is the major impediment to more widespread clinical use of this technique. Despite these barriers, human bone marrow transplantation has had important clinical application in the treatment of aplastic anemias and congenital immunodeficiency diseases and several hematological malignancies. In experimental models, work with bone marrow transplantation for the induction of tolerance to organ allografts has proved highly promising. This may provide a key for the development of treatment protocols in organ transplant recipients that would avoid or reduce the need for toxic systemic immunosuppressants.

213. The answer is A (1, 2, 3). *(Torosian, Cancer 58:1915–1929, 1986. Williams, Nutrition International 1:49–59, 1985.)* Malignant tumors require energy substrates to grow and ordinarily claim these substrates from the host. In animal studies, withholding dietary proteins diminishes the rate of tumor growth. There is no evidence in the human to suggest acceleration of tumor growth when nutritional support is provided. There is also no evidence that nutritional therapy improves the response of the tumor to therapy. For nearly a century, the association of stomach cancer and diet has been recognized. Among the wide variety of substances incriminated are nitrates and nitrosamides in food and drinking water. There is evidence that regular ingestion of vitamin C from childhood may reduce the formation of carcinogens, though reduction in the incidence of cancer has not been demonstrated. Excess amounts of dietary fat and deficiency of fiber have been clearly associated with colon cancer. Animal fats have also been associated with cancer of the exocrine pancreas, the breast, the prostate, and the endometrium.

214. The answer is A (1, 2, 3). *(Schwartz, ed 5. pp 360–361.)* Resection of metastases of lung, liver, and brain can result in occasional 5-year cures. In general, surgery should be undertaken only when the primary tumor is controlled, diffuse metastatic disease has been ruled out, and the affected patient's condition and the location of the metastasis permit safe resection. Five-year survivals as high as 18 percent have been reported for selected patients with liver metastases from colorectal primaries. However, the best results have come from resection of pulmonary metastases, in which 5-year survival rates exceed those of resection for primary bronchogenic carcinoma. Autopsy reviews have demonstrated that many patients with pulmonary metastases have no other evidence of tumor, suggesting that resectional treatment may be justified even when the lung foci are not solitary. Patient selection for pulmonary resections may be aided by measurement of tumor doubling times; patients with doubling times greater than 40 days appear to benefit most while those with doubling times less than 20 days are not significantly helped.

215–219. The answers are: 215-C, 216-A, 217-C, 218-C, 219-D. *(Recommendations for prevention of HIV transmission in health care settings. NY State J Med 88:25–31, 1988.)* Human immunodeficiency virus (HIV) has been isolated from blood, semen, vaginal secretions, saliva, tears, breast milk, cerebrospinal fluid, amniotic fluid, and urine. It is an extremely fastidious virus that ordinarily is transmitted only after repeated admixture of body fluids. Blood and semen are by far the major transmission fluids, though vaginal secretions have been weakly implicated in the transmission of HIV by epidemiologic evidence. Breast milk may be another possible mode of transmission.

220–224. The answers are: 220-E, 221-A, 222-D, 223-C, 224-B. *(Schwartz, ed 5. pp 403–412.)* Despite recent advances in tissue typing and immune modifications of graft and host, the major obstacle to successful transplantation remains rejection. Immunosuppressive regimens are required in virtually all patients. The major complications resulting from these agents are infection and bone marrow suppression.

The most recent addition to the available agents is cyclosporine A. This fungal derivative has proved, in numerous animal and human studies, to be a highly effective immunosuppressant with minimal side effects of infection. Its major clinical drawback is dose-related nephrotoxicity, which makes its use in renal transplantation difficult though still efficacious.

Azathioprine and cyclophosphamide both inhibit cell division and cause bone marrow suppression. Cyclophosphamide can cause testicular atrophy and sterility but is often substituted for azathioprine when hepatocellular damage occurs.

Antilymphocyte serum is used both prophylactically to prevent rejection, and to treat acute cellular rejection. Anaphylactoid reactions occur but are generally manageable and rarely either preclude use of the serum or lead to lethal sequelae. Thrombocytopenia is a common side effect.

Corticosteroids are used as adjuncts to all the other immunosuppressive agents listed for long-term graft maintenance and for treatment of rejection episodes. The attendant complications are well known and include, most importantly, predisposition to infection, gastrointestinal ulceration, aseptic necrosis of bone, and impaired wound healing. The recent trend toward use of substantially lower doses has led to a decrease in complications with no apparent increase in rejection rates.

Endocrine Problems and Breast

DIRECTIONS: Each question below contains five suggested responses. Select the **one best** response to each question.

225. Regarding adrenal cortical insufficiency all the following are true EXCEPT that

(A) adrenal insufficiency may be precipitated by anticoagulation with either warfarin (Coumadin) or heparin
(B) it is characteristically seen as a consequence of metastasis to the adrenal glands, especially from lung or breast
(C) adrenal insufficiency in the postoperative patient may have an insidious onset with gradually progressive hypoglycemia, hyponatremia, and hyperkalemia
(D) the most common underlying cause is prior administration of exogenous steroids
(E) the electrolyte changes of adrenal insufficiency secondary to prior chronic exogenous steroids may not occur until late in the postoperative course

226. The roentgenographic (mammographic and xeroradiographic) findings that require breast biopsy include all the following EXCEPT

(A) breast calcifications larger than 2 mm in diameter
(B) five or more clustered breast microcalcifications per square centimeter
(C) stellate-shaped breast mass
(D) breast mass with ill-defined borders
(E) dominant, well-circumscribed smooth breast mass

227. The thyroid scan shown below exhibits a pattern that is most consistent with which of the following disorders?

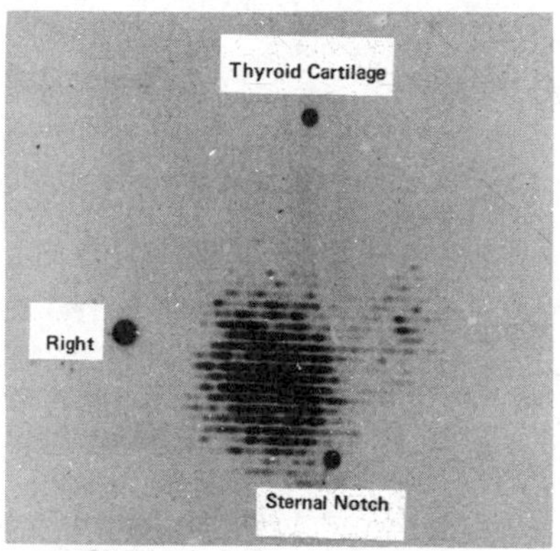

(A) Hypersecreting adenoma
(B) Graves' disease
(C) Lateral aberrant thyroid
(D) Papillary carcinoma of thyroid
(E) Medullary carcinoma of thyroid

228. A 17-year-old girl presents with an anterior neck mass. Her thyroid scan, shown below, is most consistent with which of the following disorders?

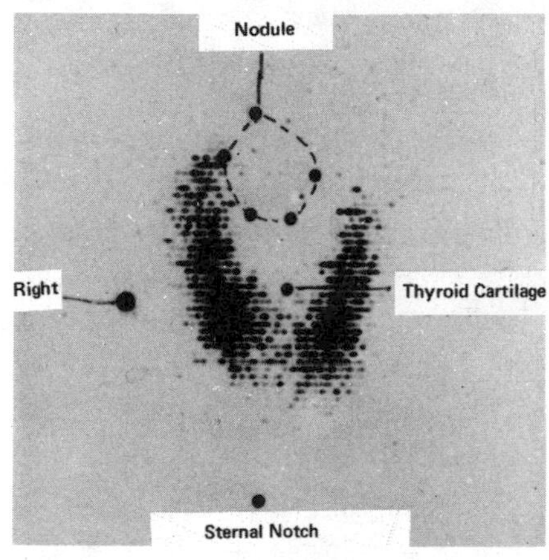

(A) Hypersecreting adenoma
(B) Parathyroid adenoma
(C) Thyroglossal duct cyst
(D) Graves' disease
(E) Carcinoma

229. The most frequent cause of primary hyperparathyroidism is

(A) idiopathic parathyroid hyperplasia
(B) familial hyperparathyroidism
(C) parathyroid adenoma
(D) primary parathyroid carcinoma
(E) ectopic production of a parathormonelike substance

230. All the following statements concerning fat necrosis of the breast are true EXCEPT that

(A) it usually is associated with a history of trauma
(B) it usually occurs in large, pendulous breasts
(C) it predisposes patients to the development of breast cancer
(D) liquefaction of fat may produce cystic spaces
(E) the treatment of choice is local excision

231. A needle-guided breast biopsy is performed for a radiographically detected cluster of microcalcifications. There is no palpable mass or axillary adenopathy. The likelihood of discovering malignant disease is

(A) less than 5 percent
(B) 10 percent
(C) 20 percent
(D) 30 percent
(E) 40 percent

232. An occult breast malignancy (ductal carcinoma) is discovered by needle-guided biopsy for clustered microcalcifications. Pathology reports that the lesion is not invasive. The patient elects to undergo an axillary lymph node dissection. The likelihood of finding at least one positive axillary node is

(A) less than 5 percent
(B) 10 percent
(C) 20 percent
(D) 30 percent
(E) 40 percent

233. An occult breast malignancy (ductal carcinoma) is discovered by needle-guided biopsy for clustered microcalcifications. Pathology reports that the lesion is frankly invasive. The patient elects to undergo an axillary lymph node dissection. The likelihood of finding at least one positive axillary node is

(A) less than 5 percent
(B) 20 percent
(C) 35 percent
(D) 50 percent
(E) 65 percent

234. All the following statements concerning Cushing's syndrome secondary to adrenal adenoma are true EXCEPT that

(A) the tumors are only rarely malignant
(B) biochemical and x-ray procedures generally make preoperative isolation of the tumors possible
(C) exploration of both adrenal glands is frequently indicated
(D) for uncomplicated tumors an abdominothoracic incision is usually employed
(E) postoperative corticoid therapy is required to prevent hypoadrenalism

235. Which statement concerning radiation-induced thyroid cancer is true?

(A) It usually follows high-dose radiation to the head and neck
(B) A patient with a history of radiation is safe if no cancer has been found 20 years after exposure
(C) Approximately 25 percent of patients with a history of head and neck irradiation develop thyroid cancer
(D) Most radiation-induced thyroid cancers are follicular
(E) The treatment of choice is a near-total (or total) thyroidectomy

236. A 32-year-old woman complains of a bloody discharge from the nipple. Physical examination reveals a small, painful, movable nodule directly beneath the areola. The nipple itself is normal. The most likely diagnosis is

(A) fibrocystic disease
(B) fibroadenoma
(C) intraductal papilloma
(D) cystosarcoma phylloides
(E) medullary carcinoma

237. The mammogram shown below exhibits findings that are most consistent with

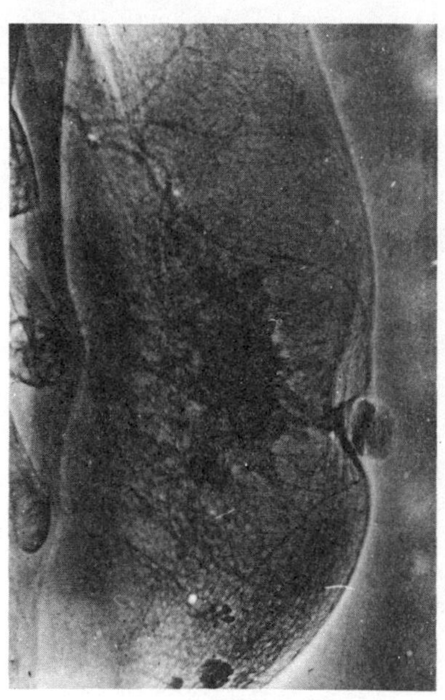

(A) fat necrosis
(B) blue dome cyst
(C) fibrocystic disease
(D) fibroadenoma
(E) carcinoma

238. The course of papillary carcinoma of the thyroid is best described by which of the following statements?

(A) Metastases are rare; local growth is rapid; erosion into the trachea and large blood vessels is frequent
(B) Local invasion and metastases almost never occur, making the term "carcinoma" misleading
(C) Bony metastases are frequent, producing an osteolytic pattern particularly in vertebrae
(D) Metastases frequently occur to cervical lymph nodes; distant metastases and local invasion are rare
(E) Rapid, widespread metastatic involvement of the liver, lungs, and bone marrow results in a 5-year survival rate of approximately 10 percent

239. A 14-year-old black girl had her right breast removed because of a large mass. The tumor weighed 1400 g and was found to have a bulging, very firm, lobulated surface with a whorl-like pattern, as illustrated below. This neoplasm is most likely to be

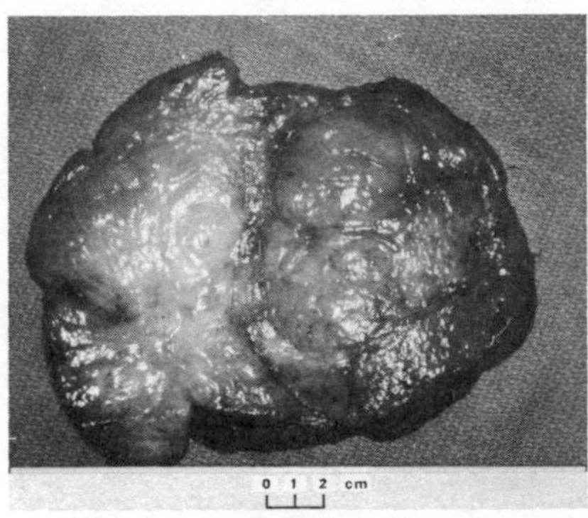

(A) cystosarcoma phylloides
(B) intraductal carcinoma
(C) malignant lymphoma
(D) fibroadenoma
(E) juvenile hypertrophy

DIRECTIONS: Each question below contains four suggested responses of which **one or more** is correct. Select

A	if	**1, 2, and 3**	are correct
B	if	**1 and 3**	are correct
C	if	**2 and 4**	are correct
D	if	**4**	is correct
E	if	**1, 2, 3, and 4**	are correct

240. Correct statements concerning Hürthle-cell carcinoma of the thyroid include which of the following?

(1) It is a form of follicular cancer
(2) It metastasizes via the blood to bone, lung, and liver
(3) Treatment consists of a near-total (or total) thyroidectomy
(4) Microscopically it consists of clusters of cells separated by areas of collagen and amyloid

241. True statements regarding Cushing's disease and syndrome include which of the following?

(1) Adrenocortical hyperplasia is the most common cause of the syndrome
(2) Overproduction of ACTH is pathognomonic of Cushing's disease
(3) The pituitary may be suppressed in the syndrome
(4) Chromophobe pituitary tumors are the cause of Cushing's disease

242. Surgically correctable forms of hypertension include which of the following?

(1) Pheochromocytoma
(2) Coarctation of the aorta
(3) Renovascular hypertension
(4) Primary hyperaldosteronism

Questions 243–245

A 65-year-old patient complains of "flushing" episodes and diarrhea. A tentative diagnosis of carcinoid syndrome is made.

243. In the patient described, a diagnosis of carcinoid syndrome would be supported by which of the following findings?

(1) Abdominal cramps
(2) A cardiac murmur
(3) Wheezing
(4) Urinary stress incontinence

244. Possible sites for an endocrinologically active tumor causing the findings in the patient described in the preceding question include the

(1) ileum
(2) bronchus
(3) cecum
(4) thymus

SUMMARY OF DIRECTIONS

A	B	C	D	E
1,2,3 only	1,3 only	2,4 only	4 only	All are correct

245. The tumor mentioned in the foregoing question is associated with which of the following characteristics?

(1) It is relatively benign, metastasizing rarely
(2) It is multiple in over 20 percent of cases
(3) The serotonin it produces is largely responsible for the characteristic clinical picture
(4) It is most frequently located in the small intestine

246. A 34-year-old woman has recurrent fainting spells induced by fasting. Her serum insulin levels during these episodes are markedly elevated. Correct statements regarding this patient's condition include which of the following?

(1) The underlying lesion is probably an alpha-cell tumor of the pancreas
(2) She should be screened for a pheochromocytoma
(3) These lesions are usually malignant
(4) Serum calcium levels may be elevated

247. Risk factors contributing to the development of breast cancer include

(1) presence of benign proliferative lesions
(2) advanced age at first pregnancy
(3) fatty diet
(4) positive family history

248. Radical neck dissection involves removal of which of the following structures?

(1) Sternocleidomastoid muscle
(2) Submandibular salivary gland
(3) Internal jugular vein
(4) Recurrent laryngeal nerve

249. Correct statements concerning subtotal parathyroidectomy include which of the following?

(1) Elevated serum calcium levels gradually return to normal over 2 to 3 weeks after surgery
(2) The two lower parathyroids are more difficult to isolate surgically than are the upper ones
(3) To avoid serious complications, surgical exploration is usually terminated as soon as an enlarged parathyroid is found
(4) The recurrent laryngeal nerve is in close proximity to parathyroid tissue and may be injured

250. Correct statements about Addison's disease include which of the following?

(1) Hyperpigmentation is a common physical sign
(2) Weight loss is almost always present
(3) Hydrocortisone administration and diet control constitute proper therapy
(4) In the United States, the disease is only rarely caused by tuberculosis

251. The incidence of breast cancer

(1) increases with increasing age
(2) has declined since the 1940s
(3) is twice as high for women 80 to 85 compared with women 60 to 65
(4) is greater among black women than white women

252. Correct statements describing medullary carcinoma of the breast include which of the following?

(1) It almost never affects the overlying skin
(2) It is frequently larger than ductal carcinoma at initial biopsy
(3) It is an aggressive neoplasm that has a worse prognosis than ductal carcinoma
(4) It is characterized by the accumulation of lymphocytes around tumor cells

253. Correct statements concerning Hashimoto's disease include which of the following?

(1) It affects females more frequently than males
(2) The involved thyroid gland often feels multinodular
(3) It is probably an autoimmune phenomenon
(4) Affected patients are usually euthyroid early in the disease

254. A 40-year-old man who has a long history of peptic ulcer disease that has not responded to medical therapy is admitted to the hospital. His serum gastrin levels are markedly elevated; at celiotomy, a small firm mass is palpated in the tail of the pancreas. Correct statements concerning this patient's condition include which of the following?

(1) Histamine or a protein meal will markedly increase basal acid secretion
(2) Secretin administration will suppress acid secretion
(3) The pancreatic mass will probably be benign
(4) Distal pancreatectomy is the treatment of choice

255. A 25-year-old woman is found to have an anterior neck mass. Her thyroid scan, shown below, exhibits findings that are consistent with which of the following disorders?

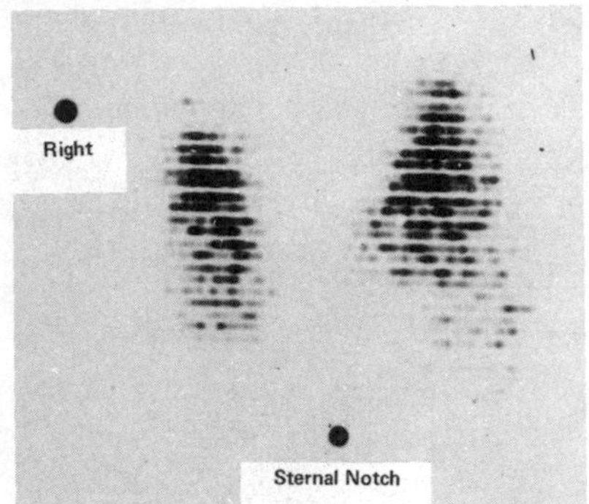

(1) Carcinoma
(2) Hyperfunctioning adenoma
(3) Follicular adenoma
(4) Graves' disease

DIRECTIONS: Each group of questions below consists of four lettered headings followed by a set of numbered items. For each numbered item select

A	if the item is associated with	(A) **only**
B	if the item is associated with	(B) **only**
C	if the item is associated with	**both** (A) and (B)
D	if the item is associated with	**neither** (A) nor (B)

Each lettered heading may be used **once, more than once, or not at all.**

Questions 256–260

(A) Graves' disease
(B) Hyperfunctioning adenoma
(C) Both
(D) Neither

256. Affected patients are usually clinically hyperthyroid

257. Thyroid scan reveals a "hot" nodule

258. Thirty to forty percent of affected patients develop cancer

259. The thyroid gland is diffusely enlarged

260. Exophthalmos is often an associated finding

Questions 261–264

(A) Hormone (estrogen and progesterone) receptor proteins
(B) Lymph node metastasis
(C) Both
(D) Neither

261. Adverse prognostic factor in breast cancer

262. Prevalent in older patients with well-differentiated breast cancers

263. Relevant to operability in breast cancer

264. Relevant to choice of adjuvant therapy in the treatment of breast cancer

DIRECTIONS: Each group of questions below consists of lettered headings followed by a set of numbered items. For each numbered item select the **one** lettered heading with which it is **most** closely associated. Each lettered heading may be used **once, more than once, or not at all.**

Questions 265–269

For each clinical description select the appropriate stage of breast cancer.

(A) Stage I
(B) Stage II
(C) Stage III
(D) Stage IV
(E) Inflammatory carcinoma

265. Tumor not palpable, clinically positive lymph nodes fixed to one another, no evidence of metastases

266. Tumor 5.0 cm, clinically positive movable ipsilateral lymph nodes, no evidence of metastases

267. Tumor 2.1 cm, clinically negative lymph nodes, no evidence of metastases

268. Tumor not palpable but breast diffusely enlarged and erythematous, clinically positive supraclavicular nodes, and evidence of metastases

269. Tumor 0.5 cm, clinically negative lymph nodes, pathological rib fracture

Endocrine Problems and Breast

Answers

225. The answer is B. *(Hardy, ed 2. pp 434–436.)* Failure to recognize adrenal cortical insufficiency particularly in the postoperative patient may be a fatal error. This error is especially regrettable because therapy (exogenous steroid) is effective and relatively easy to apply. Adrenal insufficiency may occur in a host of settings including tuberculosis (formerly the most common cause), autoimmune states, severe infections (classically, meningococcal septicemia), pituitary insufficiency, after burns, during anticoagulant therapy, and after chronic administration of exogenous steroids. Although the adrenal gland is a fairly common site for metastases, it is rare for there to be enough destruction of the glands to produce clinical adrenal deficiency. Chronic adrenal insufficiency (classic Addison's disease) should be recognizable preoperatively by the constellation of skin pigmentation, weakness, weight loss, hypotension, nausea, vomiting, abdominal pain, hypoglycemia, hyponatremia, and hyperkalemia. Death may occur within hours of surgery if a patient with Addison's disease is operated on without recognition of the adrenal insufficiency. An acute adrenal crisis involving fever, shock, and depressed mental status may occur as a response to surgery or other trauma. Patients who have adrenal insufficiency as a result of exogenous steroid therapy may not develop the classic electrolyte abnormalities until the preterminal period. Adrenal insufficiency may also develop insidiously in the postoperative period progressing over a course of several days. This insidious type tends to occur when the actual adrenal defect itself occurs in the perioperative period as would be the case with adrenal damage from hemorrhage into the gland. Measurement of blood corticosteroid levels, urinary corticosteroid secretion, urinary sodium levels, and the response to exogenous steroids is helpful in establishing the diagnosis of adrenal insufficiency.

226. The answer is A. *(Schwartz, Cancer 41:1147–1153, 1978.)* Breast biopsies have traditionally been performed to identify clinically suspicious palpable masses; also, in settings where multicentric or bilateral breast disease is likely to be encountered (e.g., lobular carcinoma), random or "blind" biopsies have been advocated by some to detect occult lesions. In more recent years the advent of screening mammography and xeroradiography has led to the discovery of nonpalpable but radiographically suspicious breast lesions that have a strong correlation with breast cancer. These clinically occult, mammographically detected lesions are (1) breast calcifications that are (a) smaller than 2 mm, (b) punctate, microlinear, or branching, (c) clustered along ducts, or (d) concentrated in clusters greater than five calcifications per square centimeter; (2) stellate-shaped lesions; (3) masses with ill-defined borders or nodular contours; (4) dominant, well-circumscribed, smooth masses that are significantly larger than any other mass in either breast; and (5) areas of increased tissue density or distorted breast architecture.

227. The answer is A. *(Sabiston, ed 13. pp 692–694.)* The thyroid scan illustrated in the question shows a single focus of increased isotope uptake, often referred to as a ''hot'' nodule; the remainder of the thyroid gland has not taken up radioactive iodine. Hyperfunctioning adenomas become independent of thyroid stimulating hormone (TSH) control and secrete thyroid hormone autonomously, resulting in clinical hyperthyroidism. The elevated thyroid hormone levels ultimately diminish TSH levels severely, thus depressing function of the remaining normal thyroid gland. An isolated focus of increased uptake on a thyroid scan is virtually diagnostic of a hyperfunctioning adenoma. Carcinomas usually display diminished uptake and are called ''cold'' nodules. Graves' disease would probably manifest as a diffusely hyperactive gland without nodularity. Multinodular goiter would display many nodules with varying activity.

228. The answer is C. *(Schwartz, ed 5. pp 1689–1690, 2118.)* The thyroid gland originates embryologically from the foramen cecum at the base of the tongue. Normally, the thyroglossal duct becomes obliterated and resorbed, but portions may remain patent and become filled with serous fluid, producing a midline cervical mass. Observe that in the scan of the patient described in the question, the mass is central and appears not to be part of the gland itself.

229. The answer is C. *(Colacchio, Head Neck Surg 2:487–493, 1980. Hardy, ed 2. pp 409–421.)* All the choices listed in the question can cause primary hyperparathyroidism. However, benign parathyroid adenoma is responsible for 85 to 90 percent of cases and hyperplasia for 8 to 12 percent. Parathyroid carcinoma, although rare, frequently produces parathormone. Ectopic production of a parathormonelike substance by oat-cell carcinomas of the lung or by renal cell carcinomas also occasionally results in primary hyperparathyroidism.

230. The answer is C. *(Schwartz, ed 5. p 562.)* Injury to breast tissue may cause necrosis of mammary adipose tissue, leading to the formation of a tender, localized, firm mass. A history of trauma is often elicited from affected patients, but less apparent factors, such as prolonged pressure, may also produce fat necrosis; half the patients in whom the diagnosis is made do not recall a history of trauma. The pathophysiology of this lesion seems to involve early development of liquefaction of mammary fat with the formation of a cystic mass. Through a process of fibrosis, this lesion evolves into a firm, sometimes calcified lump that may be difficult to distinguish from carcinoma. Excisional biopsy is usually required for definitive diagnosis; if the diagnosis of fat necrosis is confirmed, simple excision is curative.

231. The answer is D. *(Schwartz, Surg Gynecol Obstet 166:6–10, 1988.)* A recent series of 1132 biopsies for occult breast lesions that met established indications for biopsy (clustered calcifications, masses with or without calcifications, or density distortion) found a 29 percent risk of malignancy. Of these malignant lesions, 62 percent were frankly invasive. When the indication for biopsy was clustered microcalcifications (n = 594), the risk of malignancy was 31 percent.

232. The answer is A. *(Schwartz, Surg Gynecol Obstet 166:6–10, 1988.)* In a review of 1132 patients who underwent biopsy of occult breast lesions, irrespective of the specific mammographic indication for biopsy (clustered microcalcification, mass, or density distortion), no patient (n = 126) with noninvasive or microinvasive carcinoma had axillary metastasis.

233. The answer is C. *(Schwartz, Surg Gynecol Obstet 166:6–10, 1988.)* In a review of 1132 patients who underwent biopsy of occult breast lesions, 167 patients underwent axillary dissection as part of their treatment for invasive ductal or invasive lobular carcinoma. Thirty-three percent of patients had at least one positive lymph node. The incidence of positive nodes was equal whether the indication for biopsy was clustered microcalcifications or nonpalpable mass (with or without calcifications).

234. The answer is D. *(Hardy, ed 2. pp 425–436.)* A hyperfunctioning adrenal adenoma can often be palpated or visualized on x-ray. In 10 to 15 percent of cases, adenomas are bilateral, and they are occasionally malignant. To rule out multiple adenomas and to exclude malignancy it is advisable to explore both glands. The bilateral posterolateral approach avoids invasion of the peritoneal cavity and is generally less traumatic than the anterior approach, which should be reserved for complicated cases such as large or obviously malignant lesions. After tumor excision, corticosteroid therapy to correct postoperative hypoadrenalism is necessary and adrenocorticotropic hormone (ACTH), inhibited by the corticosteroid output of the autonomous tumor, returns to normal levels.

235. The answer is E. *(Hardy, ed 2. pp 395–404.)* Radiation-induced thyroid cancer was first recognized in 1950 by Duffy and Fitzgerald. It usually follows *low-dose* external radiation. Most cancers occur after exposure to 1500 rads or less to the neck, but an increase in thyroid cancer has been noted after as little as 6 rads. Salivary gland tumors and possibly parathyroid adenomas are also associated with radiation. The latent period for these tumors is 30 years or longer. Of all patients who have low-dose radiation, about 9 percent have been found to have thyroid cancer, usually of the papillary type. Treatment consists of a near-total thyroidectomy because there is a high incidence of bilaterality and because there is a greater incidence of complications if a second operation is necessary.

236. The answer is C. *(Schwartz, ed 5. pp 563–564.)* A subareolar tender lump associated with a bloody nipple discharge is a classic presentation for intraductal papilloma. Papillomas are benign proliferations of the epithelium lining the large lactiferous ducts beneath the nipple. The lesions usually are palpable as discrete, small, often tender masses, which usually are freely movable, although secondary infection and fibrosis may cause fixation to adjacent tissue. Since cancer occasionally presents with signs and symptoms indistinguishable from a ductal papilloma, excisional biopsy should always be done. If an intraductal papilloma is found, excision suffices for therapy.

237. The answer is E. *(Schwartz, ed 5. pp 555–556.)* The mammogram exhibited in the question is of an infiltrating ductal carcinoma and illustrates well the features of a malignant neoplasm. The margins of the lesion are ill-defined, indicating the infiltrative quality of the tumor. A benign neoplasm, such as a fibroadenoma, would have a discrete, pushing border rather than an indistinct infiltrating margin. Focal calcification is also present, a frequent finding in breast malignancy, and nipple retraction from tumor pressure upon lymphatics is prominently displayed. Although extremely helpful, mammography is insufficient to establish a diagnosis: excisional biopsy and histologic examination are required.

238. The answer is D. *(Hardy, ed 2. pp 395–404.)* Papillary carcinoma of the thyroid frequently metastasizes to cervical lymph nodes, but distant metastasis is uncommon. The nonaggressive nature of this tumor locally and the infrequency of distant metastases combine to produce an 80 to 95 percent 5-year survival rate. A contributing factor to the success of thyroid surgery for papillary carcinoma is the easy accessibility of cervical nodes for examination and dissection. Slow growth and a predilection for local extension are characteristics of this tumor that contribute to a high survival rate in affected persons. This is true even of patients who have limited surgery, which has led to considerable controversy regarding the extent of the indicated surgical procedure.

239. The answer is D. *(Sabiston, ed 13. pp 663–664.)* Fibroadenomas occur infrequently before puberty but are the most common breast tumors between puberty and the early thirties. They usually are well demarcated and firm. Although most fibroadenomas are no larger than 3 cm in diameter, giant or juvenile fibroadenomas frequently are very large. The bigger fibroadenomas (greater than 5 cm) occur predominantly in adolescent black girls. The average age at onset of juvenile mammary hypertrophy is 16 years. This disorder involves a diffuse change of the entire breast and does not usually manifest clinically as a discrete mass; it may be unilateral or bilateral and can cause an enormous and incapacitating increase in breast size.

Regression may be spontaneous and sometimes coincides with puberty or pregnancy. Cystosarcoma phylloides may also cause a large lesion. Together with intraductal carcinoma, it characteristically occurs in older women. Lymphomas are less firm than fibroadenomas and do not have a whorl-like pattern. They display a characteristic fish-flesh texture.

240. The answer is A (1, 2, 3). *(Hardy, ed 2. p 398.)* Hürthle-cell cancer is a type of follicular cancer, but it tends to recur more often than other types. Follicular cancer spreads hematogenously to distant sites. This is unlike papillary cancer, which metastasizes via the lymphatics. Amyloid deposits in the stroma of a thyroid tumor are diagnostic of medullary carcinoma. The treatment of choice is a near-total thyroidectomy to facilitate later body scanning for metastases and treatment with ^{131}I.

241. The answer is B (1, 3). *(Hardy, ed 2. pp 425–430.)* Cushing's disease refers to the syndrome caused by a functional pituitary tumor. Harvey Cushing first described basophilic pituitary tumors causing truncal obesity, hypertension, hirsutism, and the other characteristics of the disease. Pathologic anatomy in the adrenals is usually secondary adrenocortical hyperplasia. Primary steroid-producing adrenal or ovarian tumors may cause the syndrome, with suppression of the normal pituitary. Similar pituitary suppression may be caused by ACTH-secreting tumors elsewhere, such as oat cell lesions of the lung. Evaluation of patients has been simplified recently by availability of ACTH radioimmunoassay. Patients with both elevated 17-hydroxycorticosteroids and ACTH levels must have either a pituitary tumor (further confirmed by CT scan or MRI [magnetic resonance imaging] scan) or an occult ACTH-producing tumor in another site. Extrapituitary ACTH tumors generally are not suppressible by high-dose dexamethasone. Elevated steroid and undetectable ACTH levels eliminate the pituitary as the cause for Cushing's syndrome, placing the disorder at the level of one or both adrenals, or occasionally in ovary or testis (carcinoma, adenoma, or 1° hyperplasia).

242. The answer is E (all). *(Schwartz, ed 5. pp 1041–1059.)* All the listed conditions are correctable by surgery. Other correctable lesions are unilateral renal parenchymal disease and hyperadrenocorticism. Surgically correctable hypertension accounts for only 5 to 15 percent of the entire spectrum of this disease, but it should be carefully searched for whenever hypertensive patients are being evaluated.

243–245. The answers are: 243-A (1, 2, 3), 244-E (all), 245-C (2, 4). *(Hardy, ed 2. p 456.)* The carcinoid syndrome is characterized by flushing, wheezing, diarrhea, abdominal cramps, and the cardiac murmurs of tricuspid insufficiency and pulmonary stenosis. The syndrome is caused by vasoactive substances (including serotonin, 5-hydroxytryptophan, substance P, histamine, and kallikrein) produced by carcinoid tumors.

These tumors arise in various anatomic locations (large and small bowel, bronchus, and thymus) but from a similar embryologic origin. Although the aggressive nature of these tumors varies with location, local invasion tends to be slow with frequent metastasis. The most common location of carcinoid tumors is the small intestine; metastases, if present, tend to be hepatic.

Because the liver normally inactivates vasoactive substances produced by endocrinologically active gastrointestinal carcinoid tumors, an active lesion of this type tends to be asymptomatic until it has metastasized to the liver. While the carcinoid syndrome therefore generally implies metastatic disease, foregut carcinoids (bronchial or thymic) may produce the syndrome before metastasizing.

246. The answer is D (4). *(Hardy, ed 2. pp 454–456. Sabiston, ed 13. pp 713–715.)* Insulin-secreting *beta*-cell tumors of the pancreas produce paroxysmal nervous system manifestations that may be a consequence of hypoglycemia, although the blood glucose level may bear little relation to the severity of the symptoms, even in the same patient from episode to episode. Most insulinomas are single discrete tumors. If a careful examination of the entire gland reveals one or more specific adenomata, these can be locally excised. Excision of these tumors may be difficult because the tumors often are small and, in 10 to 15 percent of cases, multiple. Subtotal pancreatectomy is sometimes indicated to increase the probability of complete tumor removal. Patients with insulinoma may have associated ''APUD'' tumors of the pituitary and parathyroid (MEN-I). Insulinomas are not associated with MEN-II, which comprises coexistent medullary thyroid cancer, parathyroid hyperplasia, and pheochromocytoma. About one in seven of these tumors is malignant. Streptozotocin, a potent antibiotic that selectively destroys islet cells, can be useful in controlling symptoms from unresectable malignant tumors of the islet cells but probably has little to offer in the definitive management of the typical benign islet cell insulinoma.

247. The answer is E (all). *(Schwartz, ed 5. pp 556–565.)* Factors believed to increase the risk of developing breast cancer include the presence of ''proliferative'' lesions (hyperplasia, hyperplasia with atypia, sclerosing adenosis), late first pregnancy (after age 30), a diet high in animal fat, and a positive family history in the maternal lineage (that is, mother, maternal grandmother, and maternal aunts). Other identified risk factors are nationality (the lowest reported incidence is among native Japanese, the highest is among native Danes), early menarche and late menopause, previous breast carcinoma, and exposure to radiation.

248. The answer is A (1, 2, 3). *(Davis, p 1142.)* Radical neck dissection is undertaken to remove lymphatic or venous extensions, or both, of malignant neoplasms of the oral cavity, face, or neck. Typically, the procedure involves the submandibular salivary gland, sternocleidomastoid muscle, internal jugular vein, and associated adipose and lymphoid tissue. Twenty-five to thirty lymph nodes are usually recovered. Poor prognostic signs that may be disclosed by a radical neck dissection include deep invasion of local tissue, lymph node metastases, and involvement of the jugular vein. Laryngectomy also may be performed but is not technically part of the procedure. The vagus nerve and its branches are carefully isolated and preserved, unless directly involved with tumor.

249. The answer is C (2, 4) *(Davis, pp 2603–2608.)* During a subtotal parathyroidectomy, examination of more than one parathyroid is necessary to differentiate adenoma from hyperplasia since histologic examination may not be definitive. If an adenomatous parathyroid is found, the other parathyroids should be normal in size; if a hyperplastic parathyroid is found, the other parathyroids usually will be enlarged. The serum half-life of parathyroid hormone is a few hours. Following successful parathyroidectomy, serum calcium levels rapidly return to normal, usually within 1 to 2 days.

250. The answer is A (1, 2, 3). *(Davis, pp 2694–2697.)* Addison's disease, or chronic adrenal insufficiency, results from the gradual destruction of the adrenal cortex by metastatic disease, amyloidosis, various bacterial and fungal infections, certain toxic environmental pollutants, and hemorrhage into the glands from any of a wide variety of causes. Before 1950, tuberculosis was responsible for almost 90 percent of documented cases. Although the incidence of tuberculous adrenal insufficiency is much lower today, tuberculosis still accounts for almost half the cases of Addison's disease seen in the United States.

251. The answer is B (1, 3). *(Schwartz, ed 5. pp 556–565.)* Breast cancer is rarely seen before the age of 20, but thereafter its incidence increases inexorably. While the prevalence of breast cancer (the raw number of patients alive with disease) is greatest among perimenopausal women, the incidence of breast cancer (the number of new cases per 100,000 population) rises so sharply that it is twice as common among women between 80 and 85 years of age as among those 60 to 65. In addition, the age-adjusted incidence has increased steadily since the mid-1940s. Approximately one in fourteen black women will develop breast cancer; the incidence among white women is one in ten.

252. The answer is C (2, 4). *(Schwartz, ed 5. pp 564–565.)* Medullary carcinomas are characteristically soft and fleshy and usually larger than ductal carcinomas. They metastasize slowly and the prognosis is roughly five times better than in ductal carcinomas. On histologic examination, groups of lymphoid cells are associated with large nests of tumor cells. Medullary carcinomas occasionally involve the overlying breast skin and can produce fungating, ulcerated skin lesions. However, even in cases of severe dermal involvement, distant metastases may be absent.

253. The answer is A (1, 2, 3). *(Davis, pp 2533–2535.)* Hashimoto's disease, a disorder of middle-aged women, is probably an autoimmune phenomenon, and antithyroid antibodies often are demonstrable in the serum. Affected patients usually are hyperthyroid early in the disease but generally progress to a euthyroid or even hypothyroid state. Histologically, the thyroid gland contains dense aggregates of lymphocytes, and there is frank destruction of the thyroid architecture. This tissue breakdown results in local hemorrhage and fibrosis that produce firm nodular regions in the thyroid. These areas may closely mimic carcinoma on both physical examination and thyroid scan. Open biopsy is often necessary both to reach a diagnosis and to rule out carcinoma. Treatment is generally medical and consists of suppressive doses of thyroid hormone. Surgery may be indicated to relieve pressure symptoms or cosmetic problems arising from an enlarged, fibrotic thyroid gland.

254. The answer is D (4). *(Davis, pp 1444–1445, 1466–1467.)* The syndrome of a gastrin-secreting non–beta-cell pancreatic tumor is a rare entity first described by Zollinger and Ellison. They originally described a triad of (1) fulminant, complicated peptic ulceration; (2) extreme gastric hypersecretion; and (3) a non–beta-cell tumor of pancreatic islets. Over 50 percent of the tumors are malignant, and 40 percent of them have metastases at the time of surgery. Until recently, total gastrectomy had been the primary operation for this tumor; however, it is now believed that operative exploration of the patient with resection of the tumor should be done if possible. H-receptor antagonists have also proved very promising in the management of these patients. Patients with Zollinger-Ellison tumors have very high basal gastric acid (greater than 35 mEq/hr) and serum gastrin levels (usually greater than 200 pg/ml). A protein meal or histamine usually does *not* increase acid and gastrin levels as it would in conventional duodenal ulcer patients. A paradoxic *rise* in serum gastrin after intravenous secretin is diagnostic of Zollinger-Ellison syndrome.

255. The answer is B (1, 3). *(Davis, p 2553.)* The thyroid scan of the patient discussed in the question shows a discrete area of decreased radioactive iodine uptake with the remainder of the gland accepting iodine normally. This means that the tissue composing the nodule is not endocrinologically active for thyroid hormone. The two major mass lesions of the thyroid that can produce this pattern are a nonfunctioning follicular adenoma and a carcinoma. Carcinomas seldom produce thyroid hormone. Adenomas may be very active and suppress the remaining gland, but hyperactive adenomas are uncommon. Most thyroid adenomas are not hormone-producing and appear as "cold" nodules on a thyroid scan. Graves' disease produces a diffusely hyperactive gland, without nodularity. A large parathyroid adenoma could conceivably displace the thyroid gland and produce a pattern similar to the one shown, but it would be unusual. A localized infectious process also could produce such a pattern. The essential point is that a "cold" thyroid nodule may represent a carcinoma, and needle biopsy or surgical excision is indicated to rule out this possibility.

256–260. The answers are: 256-C, 257-B, 258-D, 259-A, 260-A. *(Davis, pp 2536–2542.)* Graves' disease and hyperfunctioning adenoma both result in clinical hyperthyroidism characterized by heat sensitivity, weight loss, and anxiety. The adenoma may be palpated as a discrete nodule, and it demonstrates increased uptake on radioisotope scan with functional suppression of the surrounding gland. Graves' disease produces a diffusely enlarged gland, without evidence of localized masses or nodularity.

Exophthalmos, although obscure in origin, is associated with edema and accumulation of fat and inflammatory cells in retroorbital tissues; it appears frequently in Graves' disease but rarely in a patient with hyperfunctioning adenoma.

Hyperthyroidism resulting from an adenoma is cured by excision of the adenoma. Graves' disease can be treated surgically or medically; subtotal thyroidectomy, administration of antithyroid drugs, and ablation of the thyroid with radioactive iodine all have been effective in treating this condition. Neither Graves' disease nor hyperfunctioning adenoma is significantly premalignant.

261–264. The answers are: 261-B, 262-A, 263-B, 264-C. *(Davis, pp 1275–1390. Hardy, ed 2. pp 339–364.)* Normal mammary glandular cells bind estrogen and progesterone to cytoplasmic membrane binding sites, or receptors. Breast cancers retain the ability to bind hormones to a variable degree. The older the patient and the better differentiated the tumor, the more likely the tumor is to contain a high concentration of hormone receptors. Tumors that are rich in estrogen or progesterone receptors tend to respond favorably to hormonal manipulation, usually in the form of an oral antiestrogen medication (tamoxifen). The likelihood that a tumor low or absent in hormone receptors will respond to hormonal therapy is small; these tumors have poorer prognosis than tumors that have equivalent stages in the TNM system but have high levels of receptor proteins. The status of a tumor's hormone receptors helps to guide the selection of appropriate adjuvant therapy, but does not determine a tumor's operability.

The presence of lymph node metastasis is the single most important prognostic factor in breast cancer. Tumor metastasis to even a single lymph node dramatically worsens the patient's probability of survival. Metastasis to axillary lymph nodes mandates adjuvant therapy (usually cytotoxic chemotherapy in premenopausal women, regardless of hormone receptor status, and hormonal manipulation with or without additional adjuvant therapy in postmenopausal women). Metastasis to supraclavicular or infraclavicular lymph nodes constitutes stage III disease irrespective of the size of the tumor or the presence of distant metastasis and precludes the possibility of curative surgery.

265–269. The answers are: 265-C, 266-B, 267-B, 268-E, 269-D. *(Schwartz, ed 5. pp 556–565.)* The American Joint Committee on Cancer has defined a four-tiered staging system for breast cancer based on the clinical criteria of tumor size, involvement of lymph nodes, and metastatic disease. In one version of this system, a separate category is reserved for inflammatory breast cancer. While the grouping of breast cancers into stages provides a useful shorthand for expressing a patient's survival probability, it is noteworthy that considerable heterogeneity exists both with respect to tumor size and nodal characteristics among tumors that are classified within a given stage.

The TNM stage of a breast cancer is assigned by measuring the greatest diameter of the tumor (''T''), assessing the axillary and clavicular lymph nodes for enlargement and fixation (''N''), and judging whether metastatic disease is present (''M''). In general, the worst of the three TNM parameters will determine the stage assignment.

Tumors that are not palpable are classified T0; tumors 2 cm or less, T1; tumors greater than 2 but not more than 5 cm, T2; tumors greater than 5 cm, T3; and tumors with extension into the chest wall or skin, T4.

Clinically negative lymph nodes are classified N0; positive movable ipsilateral axillary nodes, N1; fixed ipsilateral axillary nodes, N2; and clavicular nodes, N3.

Absence of evidence of metastatic disease is classified M0; distant metastatic disease, M1.

The patient in question 265 has a T0, N2, M0 lesion. This is stage III (fixed or matted nodes are a poor prognostic sign).

The patient in question 266 has a T2, N1, M0 lesion. This is stage II.

The patient in question 267 has a T2, N0, M0 lesion. Though smaller than the tumor in question 266 and without clinically involved nodes, this tumor is also stage II.

The patient in question 268 has findings compatible with inflammatory breast cancer. A biopsy of the involved skin and a mammogram would confirm the diagnosis.

The patient in question 269 has a T1, N0, M1 lesion. This is stage IV (stage IV is any T, any N, M1).

Gastrointestinal Tract, Liver, and Pancreas

DIRECTIONS: Each question below contains five suggested responses. Select the **one best** response to each question.

270. A previously healthy 15-year-old boy is brought to the emergency room with complaints of about 12 hours of progressive anorexia, nausea, and right lower quadrant pain. On physical examination, he is found to have a rectal temperature of 38.1°C (100.5°F) and has direct and rebound abdominal tenderness localizing to McBurney's point as well as involuntary guarding in the right lower quadrant. At operation through a McBurney-type incision his appendix and caecum are found to be normal, but the surgeon is impressed with the marked edema of the terminal ileum, which also has an overlying fibrinopurulent exudate. The correct procedure is to

(A) close the abdomen after culturing the exudate
(B) perform a standard appendectomy
(C) resect the involved terminal ileum
(D) perform the ileocolic resection
(E) perform an ileocolostomy to bypass the involved terminal ileum

271. A 24-year-old man is taken to the emergency room following 12 hours of nausea, vomiting, and right lower quadrant abdominal pain. He has a temperature of 38.3°C (101°F), a WBC count of 13,700/mm^3, and evidence of localized peritonitis in his right lower quadrant. At operation, his appendix is normal. The most likely cause of this man's illness is

(A) acute gastroenteritis
(B) regional enteritis
(C) Meckel's diverticulitis
(D) acute mesenteric lymphadenitis
(E) a urinary tract infection

272. A 32-year-old woman undergoes a cholecystectomy for acute cholecystitis and is discharged home on the sixth postoperative day. She returns to the clinic 2½ weeks after the operation for a routine visit and is noted by the surgeon to be jaundiced. Laboratory values on readmission show total bilirubin 5.6 mg%, direct bilirubin 4.8 mg%, alkaline phosphatase 250 IU (normal 21 to 91 IU), SGOT 52 KU (normal 10 to 40 KU), and SGPT 51 KU (normal 10 to 40 KU). An ultrasonogram shows dilated intrahepatic ducts. She undergoes the transhepatic cholangiogram seen below. Appropriate management is

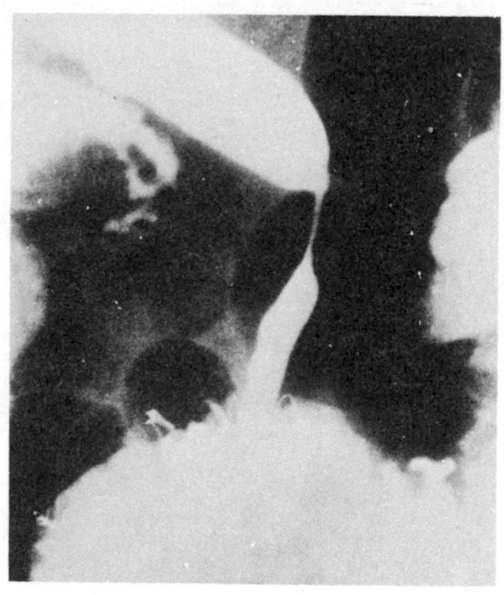

(A) choledochoplasty with insertion of a T tube
(B) end-to-end choledocho-choledochal anastomosis
(C) Roux en Y choledochojejunostomy
(D) percutaneous transhepatic dilatation
(E) choledochoduodenostomy

273. The most common presenting symptom in carcinoma of the pancreas is

(A) weight loss
(B) back pain
(C) anorexia
(D) jaundice
(E) palpable gallbladder

274. For a symptomatic partial duodenal obstruction secondary to an annular pancreas the operative treatment of choice is

(A) a Whipple procedure
(B) gastrojejunostomy
(C) vagotomy and gastrojejunostomy
(D) partial resection of the annular pancreas
(E) duodenojejunostomy

275. A 55-year-old woman with cancer of the cervix undergoes hysterectomy and is found to have pelvic lymph nodes involved with cancer. She then receives a course of external beam radiation (4500 rads). When the physician counsels her prior to her radiation treatment, she should be told of all the possible complications of radiation enteritis. These include all the following EXCEPT

(A) malabsorption
(B) intussusception
(C) ulceration
(D) fistulization
(E) perforation

276. Emergency surgery is indicated for all the following complications of ulcerative colitis EXCEPT

(A) colonic dilatation greater than 12 cm (toxic megacolon)
(B) free perforation
(C) complete intestinal obstruction
(D) intractable hemorrhage
(E) abscess formation

277. A 45-year-old executive is explored for a perforated duodenal ulcer 6 hours after onset of symptoms. He has a history of chronic peptic ulcer disease treated medically with minimal symptoms. The procedure of choice is

(A) simple closure with omental patch
(B) truncal vagotomy and pyloroplasty
(C) antrectomy and truncal vagotomy
(D) highly selective vagotomy
(E) hemigastrectomy

278. Pyogenic liver abscess is most frequently caused by

(A) generalized sepsis
(B) appendicitis
(C) diverticulitis
(D) cholangitis
(E) hepatic trauma

279. Intestinal obstruction in patients of all ages most commonly results from

(A) neoplasm
(B) intussusception
(C) inflammatory disease
(D) adhesive bands
(E) incarcerated hernia

280. All the following statements concerning carcinoma of the esophagus are true EXCEPT that

(A) alcohol has been implicated as a precipitating factor
(B) adenocarcinoma is the most common type at the cardioesophageal junction
(C) it has a higher incidence in males than females
(D) it occurs more commonly in patients with corrosive esophagitis
(E) surgical excision is the only effective treatment

281. A 63-year-old man is noted to be anemic when his physician orders routine blood tests during an annual physical examination. Stool guaiac examination is positive for occult blood. There is no history of constipation, weight loss, or abdominal pain. A barium enema is ordered and the film is pictured below. This patient should be informed that

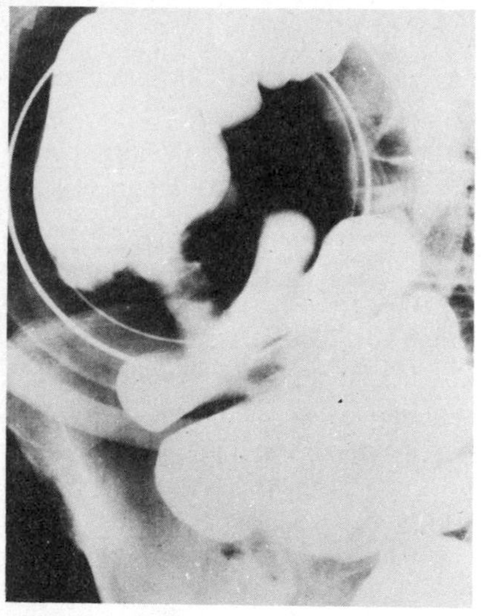

(A) his condition (anemia) is due to dietary deficiencies that need to be corrected
(B) he has diverticulosis that at this time requires no therapy
(C) he should undergo colon resection and might require a colostomy
(D) he should undergo a repeat barium enema and possibly colonoscopy in 6 months
(E) the barium enema is normal and an upper gastrointestinal series should be performed

Questions 282–283

282. A 30-year-old man with a duodenal ulcer is being considered for surgery because of intractable pain and a previous bleeding episode. Serum gastrin levels are found to be over 1000 pg/ml (normal 40 to 150) on three separate determinations. The patient should be told that the operation of choice is

(A) vagotomy and pyloroplasty
(B) highly selective vagotomy and tumor resection
(C) subtotal gastrectomy
(D) total gastrectomy
(E) partial pancreatectomy

283. Another 30-year-old man with the identical clinical situation presented in the previous question is being considered for surgery. His serum gastrin level, however, is 150 ± 10 pg/ml on three determinations. The surgeon should perform

(A) an arteriogram
(B) a secretin stimulation test
(C) a total gastrectomy
(D) a subtotal gastrectomy
(E) a highly selective vagotomy

284. The most common clinical presentation of idiopathic retroperitoneal fibrosis is

(A) ureteral obstruction
(B) leg edema
(C) calf claudication
(D) jaundice
(E) intestinal obstruction

285. A 55-year-old man who is extremely obese reports weakness, sweating, tachycardia, confusion, and headache whenever he fasts for more than a few hours. He has prompt relief of symptoms when he eats. These symptoms are most suggestive of which of the following disorders?

(A) Diabetes mellitus
(B) Insulinoma
(C) Zollinger-Ellison syndrome
(D) Carcinoid syndrome
(E) Multiple endocrine neoplasia type II

286. The most common benign tumor of the small intestine that causes clinical symptoms is

(A) lipoma
(B) fibroma
(C) leiomyoma
(D) hemangioma
(E) hamartoma

287. Massive bleeding from the lower gastrointestinal tract (distal to the ligament of Trietz) is most often caused by which of the following disorders?

(A) Meckel's diverticulum
(B) Diverticulosis
(C) Diverticulitis
(D) Ulcerative colitis
(E) Colonic carcinoma

288. A 50-year-old man presents to the emergency room with a 6-hour history of excruciating abdominal pain and distension. The abdominal film shown below is obtained. The next diagnostic maneuver should be

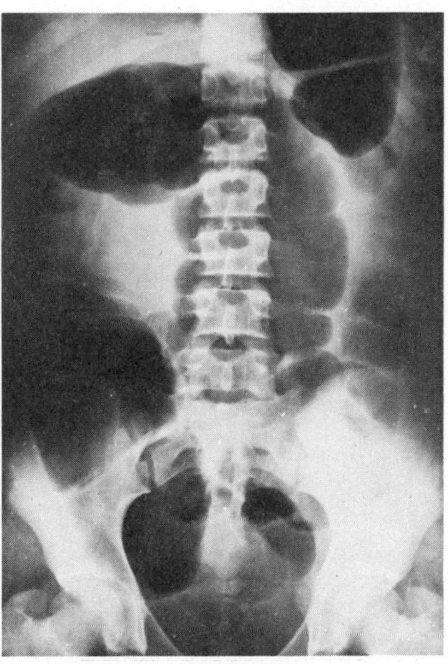

(A) emergency celiotomy
(B) upper gastrointestinal series with small bowel follow-through
(C) CT scan of the abdomen
(D) barium enema
(E) sigmoidoscopy

289. Indications for operation in Crohn's disease include all the following EXCEPT

(A) intestinal obstruction
(B) enterovesical fistula
(C) ileum–ascending colon fistula
(D) enterovaginal fistula
(E) free perforation

290. The most common malignancy of the anus is which of the following?

(A) Epidermoid (squamous) cell carcinoma
(B) Cloacogenic transitional cell carcinoma
(C) Leiomyosarcoma
(D) Melanoma
(E) Lymphoma

291. As a therapeutic modality, splenectomy might be indicated for a patient who had any of the following hemolytic disorders EXCEPT

(A) glucose-6-phosphate deficiency
(B) hereditary spherocytosis
(C) sickle cell anemia
(D) idiopathic autoimmune hemolytic anemia
(E) thalassemia major

292. A 50-year-old woman with a long history of intermittent abdominal pain caused by a documented ulcer presents with hematemesis, which is self-limited and does not require transfusion. An upper gastrointestinal series is ordered as part of her workup, and the x-ray shown below is obtained. True statements concerning this patient's condition include all the following EXCEPT

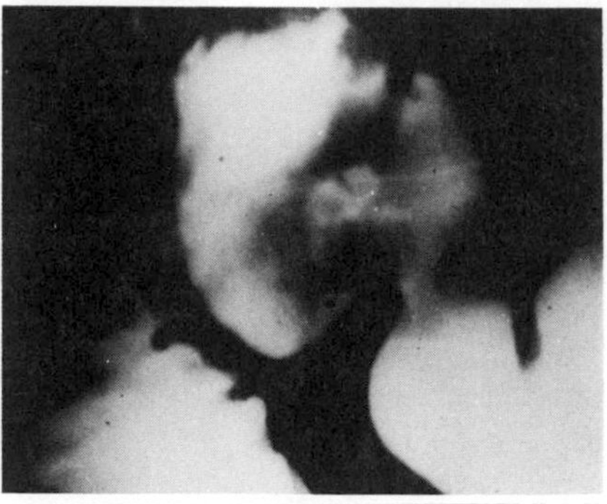

(A) it is associated with an increase in parietal cell mass
(B) it has a significant association with hyperparathyroidism
(C) affected patients often have a higher output of gastric acid than patients with gastric ulcers
(D) 70 percent of affected patients will eventually require surgery
(E) upper endoscopy is the most reliable diagnostic procedure

293. All the following statements about infantile hypertrophic pyloric stenosis are true EXCEPT that it

(A) requires correction of hypokalemic alkalosis prior to therapy
(B) usually responds to nonsurgical management
(C) frequently can be palpated
(D) is characterized by projectile vomiting
(E) affects males more commonly than females

294. All the following statements about patients with the Mallory-Weiss syndrome are true EXCEPT that

(A) they usually require surgery
(B) they usually exhibit retching or vomiting
(C) they frequently suffer from alcohol abuse
(D) they frequently have a hiatal hernia
(E) the disorder is diagnosed via endoscopy

295. The following statements concerning imperforate anus are true EXCEPT that

(A) imperforate anus affects males and females with equal frequency
(B) the rectum has descended to below the level of the levator ani muscle complex in most females
(C) the rectum usually ends in a fistulous communication
(D) the chance for eventual continence is greater when the rectum has descended to below the levator ani muscles
(E) immediate definitive repair of the anatomic defect is required to maximize the chance of eventual continence

296. Spontaneous splenic rupture is most frequently associated with which of the following disease states?

(A) Polycythemia vera
(B) Infectious mononucleosis
(C) Sarcoidosis
(D) Malaria
(E) Leukemia

297. Which of the following is the most common location for an accessory spleen?

(A) Gastrosplenic ligament
(B) Splenocolic ligament
(C) Splenic hilum
(D) Splenorenal ligament
(E) Greater omentum

298. A patient with a history of familial polyposis undergoes a diagnostic polypectomy. Which of the following types of polyps is most likely to be found?

(A) Villous adenoma
(B) Hyperplastic polyp
(C) Adenomatous polyp
(D) Retention polyp
(E) Pseudopolyp

299. In adults, the most common complication of Meckel's diverticulum is

(A) perforation
(B) bleeding
(C) obstruction
(D) intussusception
(E) carcinoma

300. Heterotopic pancreas is most commonly found in which of the following?

(A) Gallbladder
(B) Small intestine
(C) Large intestine
(D) Meckel's diverticulum
(E) Esophagus

301. A previously healthy 50-year-old woman is evaluated by her internist for intermittent crampy abdominal pain, which radiates to her back and occasionally to her shoulder and is exacerbated by eating. Workup included an upper gastrointestinal series, ultrasonogram, and oral cholecystogram. She brings the representative radiographs shown below to her surgeon. The treatment plan should be

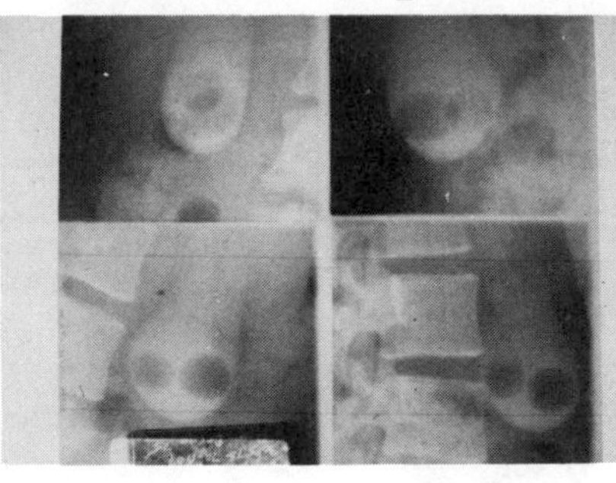

(A) reassurance and antispasmodic agents
(B) cimetidine, 300 mg, PO, qid
(C) cholecystectomy on an elective basis
(D) highly selective vagotomy
(E) chenodeoxycholic acid

302. Esophageal perforation is most likely to be caused by

(A) external trauma
(B) ingested foreign bodies
(C) instrumentation
(D) protracted vomiting
(E) carcinoma

Questions 303–304

A 60-year-old male alcoholic is admitted to the hospital with hematemesis. His blood pressure is 100/60, the physical examination reveals splenomegaly and ascites, and the initial hematocrit is 25%. Nasogastric suction yields 300 ml of fresh blood.

303. After initial resuscitation, this man should undergo

(A) esophageal balloon tamponade
(B) barium swallow
(C) selective angiography
(D) esophagogastroscopy
(E) exploratory celiotomy

304. A diagnosis of bleeding esophageal varices is made in this patient. Appropriate initial therapy would be

(A) intravenous vasopressin
(B) endoscopic sclerotherapy
(C) emergency portacaval shunt
(D) emergency esophageal transection
(E) esophageal balloon tamponade

305. A 55-year-old man complains of chronic intermittent epigastric pain and gastroscopy demonstrates a 2-cm ulcer of the distal lesser curvature. Endoscopic biopsy yields no malignant tissue. After a 6-week trial of H_2-blockade and antacid therapy, the ulcer is unchanged. Proper therapy at this point is

(A) repeat trial of medical therapy
(B) local excision of the ulcer
(C) Billroth I partial gastrectomy
(D) Billroth I partial gastrectomy with vagotomy
(E) vagotomy and pyloroplasty

306. Regarding regional enteritis, all the following are true statements EXCEPT that

(A) regional enteritis may involve any segment of the GI tract
(B) the most frequent site of involvement is the terminal ileum
(C) massive hemorrhage per rectum is common
(D) adenocarcinoma of the small bowel associated with the disease has a poor prognosis
(E) the actual cause of the disease is unknown

307. All the following findings are manifestations of the malignant carcinoid syndrome EXCEPT

(A) cutaneous flushing
(B) peripheral edema
(C) asthmatic attacks
(D) pulmonary stenosis
(E) adrenal insufficiency

308. Which of the following hernias follows the path of the spermatic cord within the cremaster muscle?

(A) Femoral
(B) Direct inguinal
(C) Indirect inguinal
(D) Spigelian
(E) Interparietal

Questions 309–310

A 70-year-old woman has signs and symptoms of small bowel obstruction. There is no history of previous surgery, but the patient has a long history of cholelithiasis for which she has refused surgery.

309. In the patient described, which of the following examinations is most likely to lead to a correct diagnosis?

(A) Barium enema
(B) Arteriogram
(C) Transhepatic cholangiogram
(D) Plain films of the abdomen
(E) Ultrasonogram of the right upper quadrant

310. Correct treatment of the woman described in the preceding question should consist of

(A) ileocolectomy
(B) cholecystectomy
(C) enterotomy and stone extraction
(D) nasogastric tube decompression
(E) intravenous antibiotics

311. Which of the following statements concerning Hirschsprung's disease is true?

(A) It is initially treated by colostomy
(B) It is best diagnosed in the newborn period by barium enema
(C) It is characterized by absence of ganglion cells in the transverse colon
(D) It is associated with a high incidence of genitourinary tract anomalies
(E) It is the congenital disease that most commonly leads to subsequent fecal incontinence

312. Esophageal atresia in combination with tracheoesophageal fistula is associated with all the following EXCEPT

(A) 80 percent survival rate following surgical repair
(B) excessive burping during feeding efforts
(C) air in the stomach
(D) copious mucus in the stomach
(E) regurgitation of feedings

313. All the following disorders are thought to involve precancerous lesions of the colon EXCEPT

(A) ulcerative colitis
(B) villous adenomas
(C) familial polyposis
(D) Peutz-Jeghers syndrome
(E) Crohn's colitis

314. Spontaneous closure of which of the following congenital abnormalities of the abdominal wall generally occurs by the age of 4?

(A) Umbilical hernia
(B) Patent urachus
(C) Patent omphalomesenteric duct
(D) Omphalocele
(E) Gastroschisis

315. All the following statements concerning desmoid tumors are true EXCEPT

(A) treatment consists of wide excision
(B) they are most often found in the abdominal wall
(C) the primary site of metastasis is local lymph nodes
(D) some tumors undergo malignant transformation to fibrosarcomas
(E) local recurrence is common

316. A 48-year-old woman develops pain of the right lower quadrant while playing tennis. The pain progresses and she presents to the emergency room later that day with a low-grade fever, a white blood count of 13,000, and complaints of anorexia and nausea as well as persistent, sharp pain of the right lower quadrant. On examination she is tender in the right lower quadrant with muscular spasm and there is a suggestion of a mass effect. An ultrasound is ordered and shows an apparent mass in the abdominal wall. Which of the following is the most likely diagnosis?

(A) Acute appendicitis
(B) Cecal carcinoma
(C) Hematoma of the rectus sheath
(D) Torsion of an ovarian cyst
(E) Cholecystitis

317. The most common malignant tumor of the liver is which of the following?

(A) Hepatoma (hepatocellular carcinoma)
(B) Hemangioma
(C) Hamartoma
(D) Angiosarcoma
(E) Metastatic neoplasms

318. Infants with anorectal anomalies tend to have other congenital anomalies. Associated abnormalities include all the following EXCEPT

(A) fistulas to the perineum or vagina
(B) fistulas to the urinary tract
(C) esophageal atresia
(D) heart disease
(E) corneal opacities

319. A patient who has acute pancreatitis is LEAST likely to have which of the following underlying disorders?

(A) Hyperparathyroidism
(B) Hypothyroidism
(C) Alcoholism
(D) Gallstones
(E) Mumps

320. A previously healthy 9-year-old child comes to the emergency room because of fulminant upper gastrointestinal bleeding. This hemorrhage is most likely to be the result of

(A) esophageal varices
(B) the Mallory-Weiss syndrome
(C) gastritis
(D) a gastric ulcer
(E) a duodenal ulcer

DIRECTIONS: Each question below contains four suggested responses of which **one or more** is correct. Select

A	if	**1, 2, and 3**	are correct
B	if	**1 and 3**	are correct
C	if	**2 and 4**	are correct
D	if	**4**	is correct
E	if	**1, 2, 3, and 4**	are correct

321. Correct statements concerning intussusception in infants include which of the following?

(1) Recurrence rates following treatment are high
(2) It is frequently preceded by a gastrointestinal viral illness
(3) A 1- to 2-week period of parenteral alimentation should precede surgical reduction when surgery is required
(4) Hydrostatic reduction without surgery usually provides successful treatment

322. Factors that contribute to the formation of an acute stress-related gastroduodenal ulcer include which of the following?

(1) Presence of acid
(2) Mucosal ischemia
(3) Breakdown of gastric mucosal barrier
(4) Foreign body irritation of the gastroduodenal mucosa

323. True statements regarding adenocarcinoma of the pancreas include that it

(1) occurs most frequently in the body of the gland
(2) carries a 1 to 2 percent 5-year survival rate
(3) is nonresectable if it presents as painless jaundice
(4) is associated with diabetes mellitus

324. A 32-year-old woman presents to the hospital with a 24-hour history of abdominal pain of the right lower quadrant. She undergoes an uncomplicated appendectomy for acute appendicitis and is discharged home on the fourth postoperative day. The pathologist notes the presence of a carcinoid tumor (1.2 cm) in the tip of the appendix. Correct statements include that

(1) the patient should be advised to undergo ileocolectomy
(2) the most common location of carcinoids is in the appendix
(3) the carcinoid syndrome occurs in more than half the patients with carcinoid tumors
(4) the tumor is an apudoma

325. A previously healthy 84-year-old man presents after 5 days without a bowel movement or flatus and complains of nausea, vomiting, and abdominal distension. The physical examination is notable only for a blood pressure of 105/60 mmHg and abdominal distension. The left-hand film is his initial upright abdominal radiograph. After proctoscopy, the right-hand film was obtained. Appropriate therapy includes

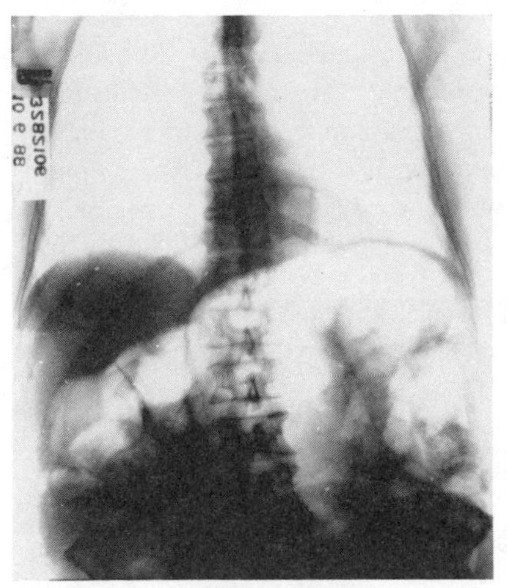

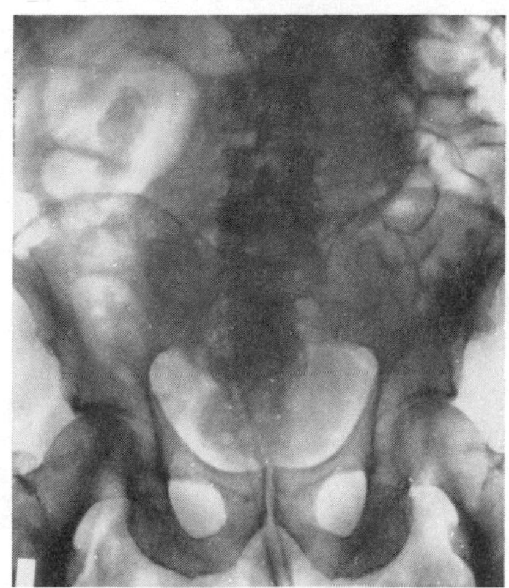

(1) emergency cecostomy
(2) removal of the rectal tube to facilitate bowel preparation
(3) preoperative irradiation of the pelvis
(4) elective resection of the sigmoid colon

---

326. A 45-year-old woman undergoes cholecystectomy and exploration of the common bile duct without complication. The T-tube study on postoperative day 10 shows three stones remaining in the common bile duct. Therapeutic alternatives include

(1) removal of stones through the T-tube tract
(2) infusion of sodium cholate through the T tube
(3) endoscopic papillotomy
(4) reoperation and biliary-enteric bypass

SUMMARY OF DIRECTIONS

A	B	C	D	E
1,2,3 only	1,3 only	2,4 only	4 only	All are correct

327. A 45-year-old alcoholic man presents to the hospital after a weekend drinking binge with abdominal pain, nausea, and vomiting. On physical examination he is afebrile and is noted to have a palpable tender mass in the epigastrium. Laboratory tests reveal an amylase of 250 U/100 ml (normal < 180). A CT scan done on the second hospital day is pictured below. Appropriate statements concerning this patient's condition include

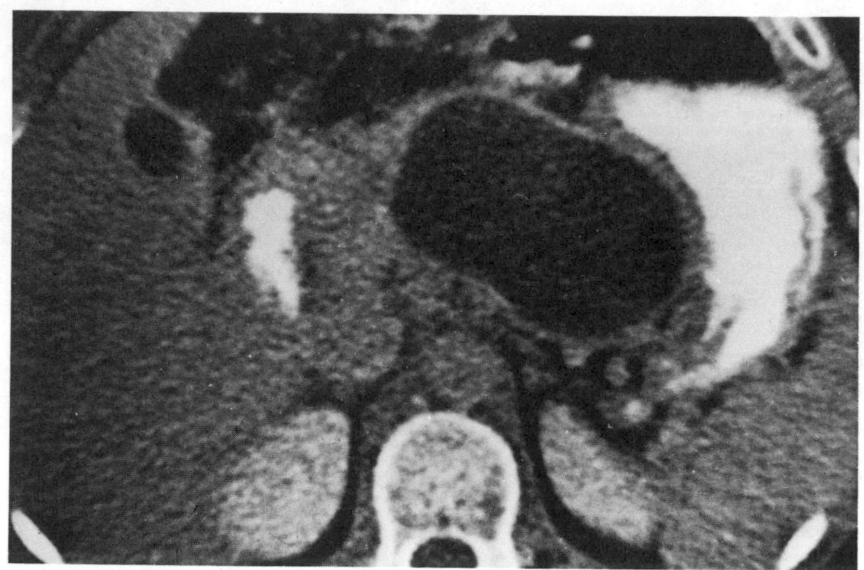

(1) the mass may result in gastric outlet or extrahepatic biliary obstruction
(2) spontaneous resolution commonly occurs
(3) the mass may be seen with acute and chronic pancreatitis
(4) the mass has an epithelial lining

328. Correct statements regarding direct inguinal hernias include that

(1) they are the most common inguinal hernias in women
(2) they protrude medial to the inferior epigastric vessels
(3) they should be opened and ligated at the internal ring
(4) Cooper's ligament repair is recommended

329. A 65-year-old woman presents with right-sided abdominal pain, which she has experienced intermittently over the last several years. On examination she has a low-grade fever and is tender in the right upper quadrant. Abdominal ultrasound is inconclusive because of overlying bowel gas. A nuclear scan with HIDA is done and is pictured below. Correct statements concerning this nuclear scan include that

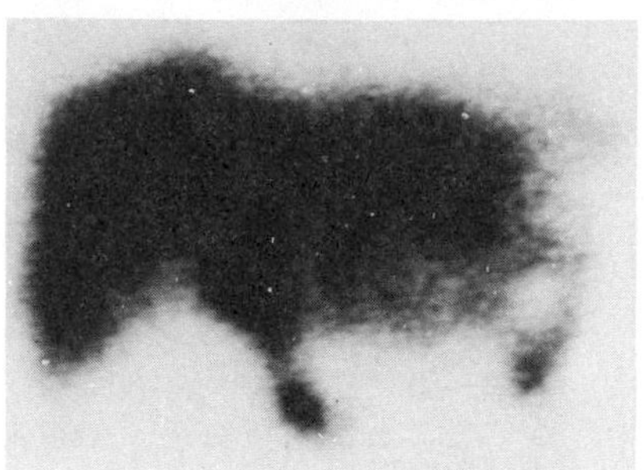

(1) it can only be done if the patient's total bilirubin is less than 5.5 mg%
(2) it relies on GI absorption
(3) it is contraindicated in patients with iodine allergy
(4) it is diagnostic of obstruction of the cystic duct

330. Correct statements regarding colorectal carcinoma include which of the following?

(1) The 5-year survival rate in patients with carcinomas limited to the bowel wall is 80 percent
(2) Chemotherapeutic agents have been of little benefit for palliation of metastatic disease, but dramatic improvement of survival rates has been noted when the agents are used as adjuvant therapy following curative resection
(3) The survival rate for patients with carcinomas of the colon has remained essentially the same for the last 30 years
(4) Radiotherapy is quite helpful in treating recurrent disease that is confined to the bowel wall

331. Superior mesenteric arterial infusion with vasopressin injection (Pitressin) to control gastrointestinal hemorrhage will

(1) decrease cardiac output
(2) decrease portal vein P_{O_2}
(3) increase systemic blood pressure
(4) be more effective than peripheral vasopressin infusion

332. An abdominal ultrasound demonstrates gallstones, and the affected patient is a good surgical risk but asymptomatic. A cholecystectomy should be performed for which of the following reasons?

(1) Increased incidence of hepatic cirrhosis
(2) Serious complications in as many as 20 percent of cases
(3) High risk of developing carcinomas
(4) Avoidance of obstruction of the common duct

333. A 28-year-old previously healthy woman arrives in the emergency room complaining of 24 hours of anorexia and nausea and lower abdominal pain that is more intense in the right lower quadrant than elsewhere. On examination she has right lower quadrant peritoneal signs and a rectal temperature of 38.3°C (101°F). At exploration through incision of the right lower quadrant, she is found to have a small contained perforation of a cecal diverticulum. True statements regarding this situation include which of the following?

(1) Cecal diverticula are acquired disorders
(2) Cecal diverticula are often solitary
(3) Cecal diverticula are mucosal herniations through the muscularis propria
(4) Diverticulectomy, closure of the cecal defect, and appendectomy are indicated

334. True statements regarding gastric polyps include which of the following?

(1) Most gastric polyps are adenomatous
(2) Patients with pernicious anemia are at particular risk to develop neoplastic gastric polyps
(3) Endoscopic removal is mandatory
(4) Adenomatous gastric polyps are premalignant lesions

335. Pancreatitis usually warrants surgical intervention in the presence of

(1) acute peritonitis
(2) severe cramping pain
(3) severe hypocalcemia
(4) common duct stones

336. The routine treatment of acute pancreatitis usually includes

(1) nothing by mouth
(2) administration of parenteral fluids
(3) administration of parenteral analgesics
(4) administration of steroids

337. Treatment of abdominal wall hernias may include

(1) expectant observation
(2) use of a corset
(3) surgical repair
(4) injection of sclerosing solutions

338. Correct statements about liver abscess include which of the following?

(1) The most common organism is *E. coli*
(2) In amebic abscess, the left lobe is involved more commonly than the right
(3) Amebic abscess is ten times more common in men than in women
(4) Tuberculosis remains a common cause

339. Correct statements concerning Zenker's diverticulum include which of the following?

(1) Dysphagia is the most common symptom
(2) Aspiration pneumonitis is likely
(3) Diagnosis is established radiographically
(4) It is a congenital lesion

Questions 340–341

A 32-year-old man undergoes a small bowel resection with primary anastomosis for intermittent small bowel obstruction secondary to a Meckel's diverticulum. On the seventh postoperative day the wound becomes tender and erythematous and the skin sutures are removed. Small bowel contents begin to drain through the wound and the diagnosis of enterocutaneous fistula is made.

340. Initial management of such a fistula requires which of the following?

(1) Skin care
(2) Volume and electrolyte replacement
(3) Control of local sepsis
(4) Proximal diversion

341. Approximately 70 percent of enterocutaneous fistulas will heal spontaneously. Which of the following will impede this healing process?

(1) Distal obstruction
(2) High volume through the fistula
(3) Foreign body
(4) Nutritional support via the enteral route

342. A patient who has a total pancreatectomy might be expected to develop which of the following complications?

(1) Diabetes mellitus
(2) Iron deficiency
(3) Malabsorption
(4) Hypophosphatemia

343. Correct statements concerning cholangitis include which of the following?

(1) The most common infecting organism is *E. coli*
(2) The diagnosis is suggested by Charcot's triad
(3) The disease occurs primarily in elderly patients
(4) Cholecystostomy is the procedure of choice in affected patients

344. Ulcerative colitis is associated with which of the following disorders?

(1) An abnormally high incidence of colonic carcinoma
(2) Sclerosing cholangitis
(3) Toxic megacolon
(4) Ocular lesions

SUMMARY OF DIRECTIONS

A	B	C	D	E
1,2,3 only	1,3 only	2,4 only	4 only	All are correct

345. Calculi are found in the common bile duct of approximately 12 percent of patients who have a cholecystectomy. Indications for exploration of the common bile duct during cholecystectomy include which of the following findings?

(1) A history of jaundice
(2) Multiple small calculi in the gallbladder
(3) Palpable calculi in the common bile duct
(4) A common bile duct that is 6 mm in diameter

346. Complications of a paraesophageal hernia include which of the following?

(1) Hemorrhage
(2) Obstruction
(3) Strangulation
(4) Reflux esophagitis

347. Diverticulosis of the colon is believed to develop as a consequence of

(1) chronic constipation
(2) an inherited predisposition
(3) a low-bulk diet
(4) tissue degeneration caused by obesity

348. Currently acceptable procedures in the elective treatment of peptic ulcer disease include which of the following?

(1) Pyloroplasty and vagotomy
(2) Parietal cell vagotomy
(3) Antrectomy and vagotomy
(4) Gastroenterostomy

349. Patients who suffer from chronic pancreatitis may be treated by

(1) pancreaticojejunostomy (Puestow procedure)
(2) distal pancreaticojejunostomy (DuVal procedure)
(3) 95 percent distal pancreatectomy
(4) lumbar sympathectomy

350. True statements concerning Meckel's diverticulum include which of the following?

(1) It is located on the mesenteric border of the ileum
(2) It is approximately 6 to 10 feet from the ileocecal valve
(3) Bleeding is the most common complication in affected adults
(4) Diverticula may contain gastric mucosa

351. A 78-year-old woman complains of lower abdominal pain and diarrhea for 2 days followed by nausea and vomiting. Physical examination is notable for a temperature of 38.89°C (102°F), atrial fibrillation with a ventricular response rate of 125/min, abdominal distension, hypoactive bowel sounds, and generalized abdominal tenderness. Laboratory tests show a white cell count of $25 \times 1000/mm^3$, BUN 58 mg/dl, and K^+ 5.2 mEq/L. Her chest radiograph is shown below. Appropriate management includes which of the following?

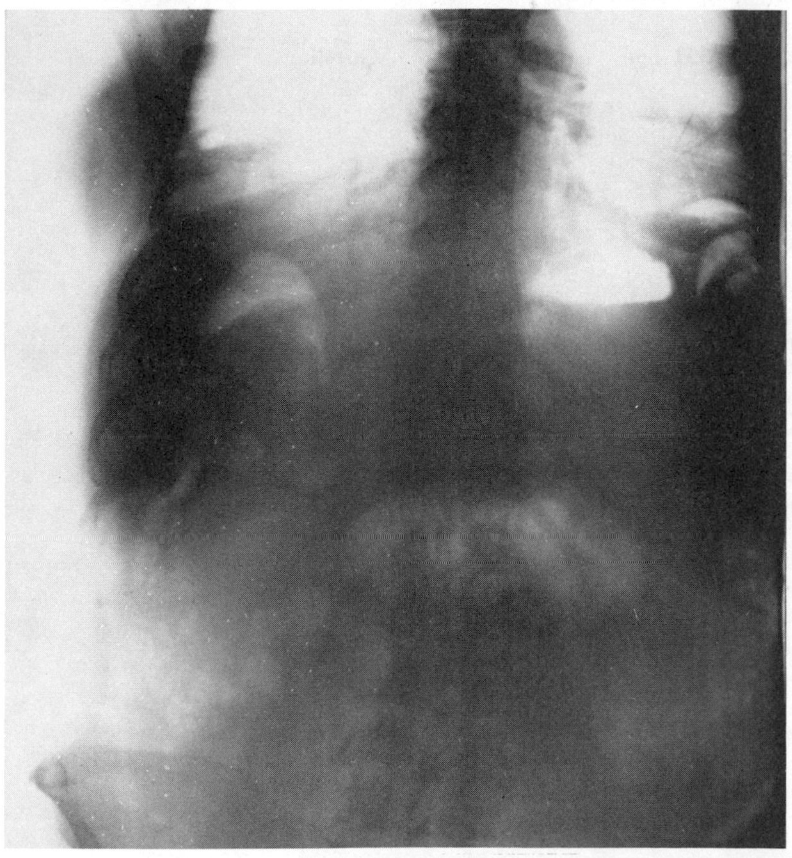

(1) Placement of a central venous catheter
(2) Colonoscopy
(3) Immediate exploratory celiotomy with prior consent for colostomy
(4) Ultrasound examination of the abdomen and pelvis

DIRECTIONS: Each group of questions below consists of four lettered headings followed by a set of numbered items. For each numbered item select

A	if the item is associated with	(A) **only**
B	if the item is associated with	(B) **only**
C	if the item is associated with	**both** (A) and (B)
D	if the item is associated with	**neither** (A) nor (B)

Each lettered heading may be used **once, more than once, or not at all.**

Questions 352–356

(A) Acute pancreatitis
(B) Chronic pancreatitis
(C) Both
(D) Neither

352. Pseudocyst formation

353. Gall stones are a common cause

354. Irreversible histopathology

355. Endoscopic retrograde cholangiopancreatography (ERCP)

356. Risk factor for adenocarcinoma of the pancreas

Questions 357–361

(A) Ulcerative colitis
(B) Crohn's disease (Crohn's colitis)
(C) Both
(D) Neither

357. Transmural disease

358. Risk factor for colon cancer

359. Megacolon

360. Perianal fistulas

361. Colonoscopy contraindicated

DIRECTIONS: Each group of questions below consists of lettered headings followed by a set of numbered items. For each numbered item select the **one** lettered heading with which it is **most** closely associated. Each lettered heading may be used **once, more than once, or not at all.**

Questions 362–365

Match each sign below with the appropriate disorder.

(A) Acute cholecystitis
(B) Acute pancreatitis
(C) Acute cholangitis
(D) Splenic rupture
(E) Pancreatic cancer

362. Kehr's sign

363. Murphy's sign

364. Cullen's sign

365. Courvoisier's sign

Questions 366–370

For each statement below, select the hernia with which it is most closely associated.

(A) Direct inguinal hernia
(B) Umbilical hernia
(C) Sliding hernia
(D) Femoral hernia
(E) Omphalocele

366. Recurrence is most likely following repair

367. A viscus makes up one wall of the hernia sac

368. If asymptomatic, does not require repair in young children

369. Viscera is covered only by peritoneum

370. Diagnosis often is difficult

Questions 371–374

Match the following.

(A) Rupture of the diaphragm
(B) Paraesophageal hiatus hernia
(C) Sliding hiatus hernia
(D) Foramen of Bochdalek hernia
(E) Foramen of Morgagni hernia

371. The most common congenital diaphragmatic hernia in infants

372. The hernia most likely to cause acute respiratory distress in infants

373. A very common defect in adults; frequently associated with gastroesophageal reflux

374. A congenital hernia that is most frequently discovered as an incidental finding in adults

Gastrointestinal Tract, Liver, and Pancreas

Answers

270. The answer is B. *(Schwartz, ed 5. p 1201.)* Patients with regional enteritis usually have a chronic and slowly progressive course with intermittent symptom-free periods. The usual symptoms are anorexia, abdominal pain, diarrhea, fever, and weight loss. There are extraintestinal syndromes that may be seen with the disease such as ankylosing spondylitis, polyarthritis, erythema nodosum, pyoderma gangrenosa, gallstones, hepatic fatty infiltration, and fibrosis of the biliary tract, pancreas, and retroperitoneum. However, in about 10 percent of patients, especially those who are young, the onset of the disease is abrupt and may be mistaken for acute appendicitis. Appendectomy is indicated in such patients as long as the caecum at the base of the appendix is not involved, otherwise the risk of fecal fistula must be considered. Interestingly, about 90 percent of patients who present with the acute appendicitislike form of regional enteritis will not progress to develop the full-blown chronic disease. Thus, resection or bypass of the involved areas is not indicated at this time.

271. The answer is D. *(Schwartz, ed 5. pp 1319–1321, 1513–1514.)* The presentation of symptoms, physical findings, and laboratory data in the question is classically associated with acute appendicitis. However, this syndrome may be mimicked by all the alternative disorders listed as well as by several others. The accepted accuracy of diagnosis for acute appendicitis should be about 80 to 85 percent; because many of the other disorders require surgical intervention, none is adversely affected by operative exploration. When acute appendicitis is not found, the differential diagnosis in descending order of frequency includes acute mesenteric lymphadenitis, acute pelvic inflammatory disease, twisted ovarian cyst or ruptured graafian follicle, and acute gastroenteritis. Other less common causes include Meckel's diverticulitis, regional enteritis, urinary tract infection, ureteral stone, *Yersinia* infection, intussusception, ruptured ectopic pregnancy, perforated ulcer, and perforating cecal carcinoma, among others. It is imperative that the surgeon perform a thorough exploration to determine the cause of the patient's illness once appendicitis has been ruled out.

272. The answer is C. *(Sabiston, ed 13. p 1134.)* The scenario in the question is a typical course of a patient with iatrogenic common bile duct injury. These injuries commonly occur in the proximal portion of the extrahepatic biliary system. The transhepatic cholangiogram documents a biliary stricture, which in this clinical setting is best dealt with surgically. Choledochoduodenostomy generally cannot be performed because of the proximal location of the stricture. The best results are achieved with end-to-side choledochojejunostomy (Roux en Y) performed over a stent. Percutaneous transhepatic dilatation has been attempted in select cases, but follow-up is too short to make an adequate assessment of this technique. Primary repair of the common bile duct may result in recurrent stricture.

273. The answer is A. *(Schwartz, ed 5. p 1430.)* Weight loss is the most common symptom in carcinoma of the pancreas, no matter where the lesion is located. Pain is a frequent symptom, present in 70 to 80 percent of the cases. Jaundice will appear in about three-quarters of the patients with tumors in the head of the pancreas and a palpable gallbladder is present in only about one-half of these cases. Anorexia occurs in about half the cases of pancreatic cancer.

274. The answer is E. *(Schwartz, ed 5. p 1415.)* A bypass procedure is the operation of choice for obstruction secondary to an annular pancreas. A Whipple procedure is too radical a therapy for this benign disease and a partial resection of the annular pancreas often is complicated by fistula. Duodenojejunostomy is much more physiologic than gastrojejunostomy and does not require a vagotomy to prevent marginal ulceration; it is therefore the procedure of choice.

275. The answer is B. *(Sabiston, ed 13. pp 962–966.)* The effects of radiation on the intestine depend on a variety of factors, which include the age of the patient, temperature, degree of oxygenation, and metabolic activity. Acute intestinal radiation injury is manifested in the bowel by the cessation of viable cell production and is seen clinically as diarrhea or gastrointestinal bleeding. Progressive vasculitis and fibrosis are seen in the latter stages of radiation injury and may result in malabsorption, ulceration, fistulization, or perforation. Intussusception is generally not associated with radiation injury.

276. The answer is E. *(Schwartz, ed 5. pp 1237–1242.)* Ulcerative colitis requires surgical management in only approximately 20 to 25 percent of affected patients, and even in these cases the surgery usually is elective. However, emergency surgical intervention does become necessary in the presence of toxic megacolon, total intestinal obstruction, uncontrollable hemorrhage, and free perforation with peritonitis. Occasionally, a localized perforation leads to an abscess. This condition generally can be treated by elective surgery after the affected patient has been stabilized. Colonic dilatation of less than 12 cm probably should be initially treated by medical means.

277. The answer is C. *(Sabiston, ed 13. pp 829–830.)* Perforation of a duodenal ulcer is an indication for emergency celiotomy and closure of the perforation. In patients with no prior history of peptic ulcer disease, simple closure with an omental patch is recommended. Seventy-two percent of patients who are asymptomatic preoperatively will remain so postoperatively. Patients with long-standing ulcer disease require a definitive acid-reducing procedure, except in high-risk situations. The choice of procedure is made by weighing the risk of recurrence against the incidence of undesirable side effects of the procedure, and considerable controversy persists about this issue. Antrectomy and truncal vagotomy offers a recurrence rate of 1 percent, but carries a 15 to 25 percent incidence of sequelae such as diarrhea, dumping syndrome, bloating, and gastric stasis. Highly selective vagotomy, if technically feasible, offers a 1 to 5 percent incidence of side effects but carries a recurrence rate of 10 to 13 percent in some series, although results are better when gastric and prepyloric ulcers are excluded. In general, definitive acid-reducing procedures should be postponed if the perforation is more than 12 hours old, or if there is extensive peritoneal soilage. Pyloroplasty and truncal vagotomy carries intermediate rates of recurrence and side effects, but has the advantage of speed in the setting of very ill patients with acute perforation.

278. The answer is D. *(Schwartz, ed 5. pp 1335–1336.)* All conditions listed in the question may result in pyogenic liver abscess. Although, in the past, appendicitis was the principal cause, cholangitis is currently the most likely cause. Treatment consists of surgical or percutaneous catheter drainage. For the patient with a large solitary abscess, which is properly drained, the prognosis is good. There remains, however, a substantial mortality associated with multiple abscess formation.

279. The answer is D. *(Schwartz, ed 5. pp 1074–1076.)* The mechanisms of mechanical small bowel obstruction may be described as (1) obstruction of the lumen; (2) encroachment of the lumen by an intrinsic process of the bowel wall; and (3) compression of the lumen by a process extrinsic to the bowel. The classifications of obstruction based on clinical and pathologic findings are as follows: (1) simple mechanical obstruction without vascular compromise; (2) strangulation obstruction in which the mesenteric vessels to the obstructed segment are occluded; and (3) closed-loop obstruction in which both the proximal and distal limbs of the involved loop are blocked. Causes of intestinal obstruction range from fecal impaction to radiation stricture. However, combining all age groups, currently the most frequent cause of obstruction is adhesive bands. Incarcerated inguinal hernia is next, followed by neoplasms. These three entities account for more than 80 percent of all obstructions. The frequency varies for different age groups; hernia is by far the most common cause in childhood, whereas neoplasm and diverticulitis are the most frequent causes in the elderly.

280. The answer is E. *(Sabiston, ed 13. pp 737–746.)* Carcinoma of the esophagus occurs primarily in the sixth and seventh decades of life in a male:female ratio of 3:1. Although the cause is unknown, alcohol, tobacco, and dietary factors have been implicated as causative agents. A high incidence is reported in patients with corrosive esophagitis. The malignant tumors arising in the esophagus usually are squamous cell carcinomas except those involving the esophagogastric junction, which usually are adenocarcinomas. Even though squamous cell carcinomas are weakly radiosensitive, surgical extirpation affords reasonable, if short-term, palliation. Some authorities recommended radiotherapy for palliation alone or in combination with surgery to treat this lesion. Adenocarcinomas are not particularly radiosensitive and surgical treatment is generally employed. Following resection for esophageal carcinoma among the highly select group of patients whose tumors are still resectable when the diagnosis is made, survival is only about 14 percent at 5 years. The overall 5-year survival is under 5 percent.

281. The answer is C. *(Schwartz, ed 5. pp 1270–1279.)* The barium enema depicted in the question demonstrates an apple-core lesion of the ascending colon, which is most consistent with an adenocarcinoma. This patient requires resection of the lesion in an attempt to cure the carcinoma and to avoid further bleeding. The location of the lesion makes colostomy an unlikely possibility, but the patient should be informed that a stoma (either temporary or permanent) is always a possibility in colon surgery. Left-sided lesions in the rectosigmoid or rectum make the need for colostomy much more likely.

282–283. The answers are: 282-B, 283-B. *(Schwartz, ed 5. pp 1436–1437.)* Total gastrectomy was formerly the procedure of choice for patients with Zollinger-Ellison syndrome (ZES). However, with the knowledge that most patients will die of metastatic disease and that symptoms can often be controlled with H_2-receptor antagonists, the role for surgery has changed. Initial surgical exploration is aimed at curative resection of the tumor. Unfortunately metastatic disease is often present or will develop at a later date despite tumor resection. Therefore, highly selective vagotomy is also added to the procedure to reduce the required dose of H_2-receptor antagonists. The second patient has a gastrin level suggestive of but not diagnostic of ZES. A secretin stimulation test will cause a significant rise in serum gastrin levels in patients with ZES.

284. The answer is A. *(Schwartz, ed 5. pp 1518–1519.)* Idiopathic retroperitoneal fibrosis is a nonsuppurative inflammatory process of the retroperitoneum that causes problems by extrinsic compression of retroperitoneal structures. The ureters, aorta, and inferior vena cava are most at risk; however, the aorta is quite resistant to compression and the inferior vena cava has multiple collaterals so that ureteral obstruction is the most common presentation of this disease process. The common bile duct and duodenum may be compressed and obstructed, but this occurs much less frequently. Treatment of ureteral obstruction includes conservative therapy with steroids. Often surgical intervention is required and ureterolysis with intraperitoneal transplantation is the current procedure of choice. Biopsies must also be taken to exclude a malignant process as the cause of the fibrosis.

285. The answer is B. *(Schwartz, ed 5. pp 1434–1435.)* Tumors arising from the pancreatic beta cells give rise to hyperinsulinism. Seventy-five percent of these tumors are benign adenomas and in fifteen percent of affected patients the adenomas are multiple. Symptoms relate to a rapidly falling blood glucose level and are due to epinephrine release triggered by hypoglycemia (sweating, weakness, tachycardia). Cerebral symptoms of headache, confusion, visual disturbances, convulsions, and coma are due to glucose deprivation of the brain. Whipple's triad summarizes the clinical findings in patients with insulinomas: (1) attacks precipitated by fasting or exertion; (2) fasting blood glucose concentrations below 50 mg/100 ml; (3) symptoms relieved by oral or intravenous glucose administration. These tumors are treated surgically and simple excision of an adenoma is curative in the majority of cases.

286. The answer is C. *(Schwartz, ed 5. p 1205.)* Benign tumors of the small intestine are rare and are generally asymptomatic. When they become clinically apparent they present with occult bleeding or obstruction. The leiomyoma is the most common tumor that causes symptoms, closely followed by the lipoma. Adenomas are the most frequent tumor in autopsy series. Management involves resection of the small bowel with primary anastomosis.

287. The answer is B. *(Schwartz, ed 5. pp 1090–1091.)* Blood passed per rectum is caused most often by bleeding that originates in the upper gastrointestinal tract. However, in bleeding that does originate from lesions distal to the ligament of Trietz, colonic carcinoma is the most common cause of bloody stools. Diverticulosis is the most common cause of massive lower gastrointestinal bleeding. Meckel's diverticulum, diverticulitis, and ulcerative colitis are all less common causes of rectal bleeding. When occult or gross blood is found in stools, carcinoma of the colon must be ruled out.

288. The answer is E. *(Schwartz, ed 5. pp 1262–1263.)* The film shows a markedly distended colon. The differential diagnosis includes tumor, foreign body, and colitis, but by far more likely is either cecal or sigmoid volvulus. Sigmoid volvulus may be ruled out quickly by proctosigmoidoscopy, which is preferable to barium enema, since sigmoid volvulus may be treated successfully by rectal tube decompression via the sigmoidoscope. If sigmoidoscopy is negative, the working diagnosis, based on this classic film, must be cecal volvulus; barium enema would clinch the diagnosis, but the colon might rupture in the intervening 1 to 2 hours. Emergency celiotomy should be done.

289. The answer is C. *(Schwartz, ed 5. pp 1200–1202.)* Surgical treatment of Crohn's disease is aimed at correcting complications that are causing symptoms. Intestinal obstruction is usually partial and secondary to a fixed stricture that is not responsive to anti-inflammatory agents. When the obstruction causes symptoms that compromise nutritional status, surgery is warranted. Fistula formation in itself is not an indication for surgery. Fistulas between the intestine and the bladder and the intestine and the vagina, however, generally cause significant symptoms and warrant surgical intervention, while an ileum–ascending colon fistula is very common yet rarely symptomatic. Perforation of bowel into the free abdominal cavity is obviously a surgical emergency.

290. The answer is A. *(Schwartz, ed 5. pp 1289–1292.)* The two common varieties of anal carcinoma are squamous cell carcinoma and transitional cell carcinoma. Metastatic spread is to the superior rectal nodes, pelvic nodes, and inguinal nodes. Therapy is initially combined radiotherapy and chemotherapy (Nigro protocol) followed by local excision or abdominoperineal resection if residual tumor is present. The anal canal is the third most common site for melanomas (after skin and eyes). Lymphomas and leiomyosarcoma are extremely rare in this location.

291. The answer is A. *(Schwartz, ed 5. pp 1447–1452.)* In hemolytic, thrombocytopenic, or leukopenic disorders, splenectomy is generally employed after failure of other methods of treatment. The attitude toward splenectomy is being reassessed in many cases owing to recently documented late postoperative complications of sepsis and thromboembolism. However, when the procedure is employed appropriately, the benefit may be dramatic. Blood dyscrasias in which splenectomy has been a successful therapeutic measure in selected circumstances include hereditary spherocytosis, hereditary elliptocytosis, pyruvate kinase deficiency, thalassemia major, sickle cell anemia, idiopathic autoimmune hemolytic anemia, idiopathic thrombocytopenic purpura, thrombotic thrombocytopenic purpura, primary hypersplenism, Felty's syndrome, and Gaucher's disease. It has not proved to be of any value in patients suffering from glucose-6-phosphate deficiency and there is no rationale for splenectomy in this disorder.

292. The answer is D. *(Schwartz, ed 5. pp 1169–1173.)* The x-ray presented in the question demonstrates a duodenal ulcer for which surgery was recommended. About 2 percent of the population suffers from duodenal ulcer but surgical management is rarely necessary with contemporary techniques of medical management. Indications for surgery for duodenal ulcer include obstruction, perforation, hemorrhage, and intractability. About 20 percent of patients with duodenal ulcer eventually require surgery.

293. The answer is B. *(Schwartz, ed 5. pp 1698–1699.)* Hypertrophic pyloric stenosis affects males more commonly than females and usually presents with the onset of projectile vomiting in an infant 3 to 10 weeks of age. The enlarged pyloris often can be palpated in the right upper abdomen as a mass the size and shape of an olive. Treatment consists of correction of any electrolyte imbalance that may have resulted from prolonged vomiting, followed by division of the seromuscular layer of the pylorus to allow herniation of the mucosa (pyloromyotomy). Peptic ulcer would be extremely unusual in infancy and jejunal atresia would present problems before 3 weeks of age. Antral and duodenal webs are considerably less common than pyloric stenosis.

294. The answer is A. *(Schwartz, ed 5. p 1180. Todd, Ann Surg 186:146–148, 1977.)* The lesions associated with the Mallory-Weiss syndrome are described as longitudinal mucosal tears along the gastroesophageal junction caused by increased intraabdominal pressure. Any cause of increased intraabdominal pressure (e.g., vomiting, retching, external forces applied to the abdomen) can cause this lesion, which presents as painless upper gastrointestinal bleeding. Endoscopy is helpful in establishing the diagnosis and is the procedure of choice. Many authors have noted an association of the Mallory-Weiss syndrome with hiatal hernia and alcohol abuse, but neither is an essential component. About 75 percent of these patients will cease bleeding without invasive therapeutic maneuvers (i.e., surgery or angiographic embolization).

295. The answer is E. *(Schwartz, ed 5. pp 1708–1709.)* Imperforate anus affects males and females with equal frequency, occurring in 1 of each 20,000 live births. It is due to failure of descent of the urorectal septum. Imperforate anus may be broadly classified into "high" or "low," depending on whether the rectum ends above or below the level of the levator ani complex. In 90 percent of females, but only 50 percent of males, the lesion is of the low variety. The rectal fistula may end in the prostatic urethra or vagina in the high cases, while the low cases terminate in a perineal fistula. For the low cases, only a perineal operation may be required and these children will be expected to be continent. A pull-through procedure will be required for the high imperforate anus and the chances for continence are less. If there is doubt about the level or location of the termination of the rectum, it is better to perform a colostomy than to compromise chances of continence by an injudicious perineal approach.

296. The answer is D. *(Schwartz, ed 5. p 1446.)* Spontaneous rupture of the spleen is a rare event and almost always occurs in conjunction with a diseased spleen. A history of minor trauma, which may not originally have been appreciated, can usually be elicited in these cases. Malaria is the most common disease state associated with spontaneous splenic rupture. Infectious mononucleosis is a close second behind malaria and in the United States is the most commonly associated disease state. Spontaneous splenic rupture may also be seen in conjunction with leukemia, sarcoidosis, polycythemia vera, hemolytic anemia, congestive splenomegaly, and splenic abscess.

297. The answer is C. *(Schwartz, ed 5. p 1441.)* Accessory spleens are present in 15 to 30 percent of patients. These organs obtain their blood supply from the splenic artery. Accessory spleens may be found in the gastrosplenic ligament, the splenocolic ligament, the splenorenal ligament, the greater omentum, the gastrocolic ligament, the female pelvis, and the scrotum. They are most commonly found, however, in the splenic hilum.

298. The answer is C. *(Schwartz, ed 5. pp 1264–1268.)* Varying types of colonic polyps can be distinguished on pathologic examination. Adenomatous polyps are distributed throughout the entire large bowel, more commonly in the right and left colon than the rectum. They are often pedunculated and show an increased number of glands compared with normal mucosa. Although polyps that appear in familial polyposis are indistinguishable from single adenomatous polyps, they are manifested much earlier in life. Carcinomatous changes in patients who have familial polyposis occur approximately 20 years before carcinomatous changes of the bowel occur among patients in the general population.

299. The answer is C. *(Schwartz, ed 5. p 1212.)* Meckel's diverticulum is the most common diverticulum of the small bowel. It is located on the antimesenteric border, usually within 3 feet of the ileocecal valve. The condition is frequently asymptomatic; symptoms that do occur usually are apparent during childhood. Complications in adults include obstruction, bleeding, perforation, and pain that closely mimics that of appendicitis. Carcinoma and intussusception, although rare complications of Meckel's diverticulum, may arise in elderly persons and children, respectively.

300. The answer is D. *(Schwartz, ed 5. p 1415.)* Heterotopic or accessory pancreas refers to an area of ectopic pancreatic tissue. This tissue is located in a submucosal position and is generally between 2 and 4 mm in size. It is most commonly found in the stomach or in a Meckel's diverticulum and can be confused with a leiomyoma or an ulcer.

301. The answer is C. *(Schwartz, ed 5. p 1398.)* This patient has symptomatic cholelithiasis. In view of her symptoms, her relatively young age, and documented calculi, she should undergo an elective cholecystectomy to alleviate symptoms and prevent cholecystitis and choledocholithiasis (and/or cholangitis). Selective vagotomy is a treatment for peptic ulcer disease (as is cimetidine). Chenodeoxycholic acid has been demonstrated to dissolve radiolucent stones completely in 13.5 percent and partially in 41 percent of patients so treated. Recurrence of cholelithiasis is quite likely following discontinuation of treatment, and therefore cholecystectomy remains the most effective therapy.

302. The answer is C. *(Sabiston, ed 13. pp 749–752. Schwartz, ed 5. pp 1145–1147.)* While all the conditions listed in the question can cause perforation of the esophagus, the most common cause is iatrogenic, i.e., some form of esophageal instrumentation (esophagoscopy, intubation, dilation). The most common site of perforation, regardless of cause, is just proximal to the cricopharyngeal muscle at the introitus of the esophagus. The second most common site is just above the esophagogastric junction. Perforations in the body of the esophagus are relatively infrequent.

303–304. The answers are: 303-D, 304-B. *(Sabiston, ed 13. pp 1100–1116.)* The diagnosis of bleeding esophageal varices is aided in the adult by stigmata of portal hypertension. Upper gastrointestinal hemorrhage in cirrhotics is due to esophageal varices in less than half of patients. Gastritis and peptic ulcer disease account for the majority of cases. Esophagoscopy is the single most reliable means of establishing the source of bleeding, though variations in transvariceal blood flow may result in nonvisualization of the varices. In addition, endoscopic sclerotherapy is reported to control acute variceal hemorrhage in 80 to 90 percent of cases and carries an acute mortality lower than other procedures. Barium swallow has a high false negative rate and offers no therapeutic advantage. Celiac angiography will rule out arterial hemorrhage and will demonstrate venous collateral circulation, but will not demonstrate variceal bleeding. Parenteral vasopressin controls variceal hemorrhage by constriction of the splanchnic arteriolar bed and a resultant drop in portal pressure. Intraarterial vasopressin offers no advantage over intravenous administration and requires a mesenteric catheter. The reported control rate is 50 to 70 percent. Esophageal balloon tamponade controls variceal hemorrhage in two-thirds of patients, but may also control bleeding ulcers and thereby obscure the diagnosis. Although balloon tamponade has reduced the mortality and morbidity from variceal hemorrhage in good-risk patients, increasing awareness of associated complications (aspiration, asphyxiation, and ulceration at the tamponade site), as well as a rebleeding rate of 40 percent, has reduced its use. It is indicated as a temporary measure when vasopressin and sclerotherapy fail. Emergency portacaval shunt is advised in good-risk cirrhotic patients whose bleeding is not controlled with vasopressin or sclerosis. The mortality for patients with bleeding varices not subjected to shunting is between 66 and 73 percent, whereas operative mortality of emergency shunts ranges from 20 to 50 percent. Esophageal transection with the autostapler carries the same mortality as shunt procedures and the rebleeding rate is estimated to be 50 percent at 1 year.

305. The answer is C. *(Thomas, Ann Surg 195:189–195, 1982.)* Benign gastric ulcers have a peak incidence in the fifth decade, with male predominance. About 95 percent of gastric ulcers are located near the lesser curvature. It should be recognized that up to 16 percent of patients with gastric carcinoma pass a 12-week healing trial and that benign ulcers may enlarge during medical therapy. Therefore, the possibility of malignancy must be assessed by biopsy despite a 5 to 10 percent false negative rate. Six weeks of medical therapy will heal many gastric ulcers, but a recurrence rate as high as 63 percent and the serious consequence of complications in this older group of patients warrant surgery for recurrent or nonhealing ulcers. A distal gastrectomy with gastroduodenostomy is usually feasible in the absence of duodenal disease. Vagotomy, while advocated by some, is generally not included. Local excision with definitive distal resection or vagotomy and pyloroplasty is appropriate for a proximal ulcer that would otherwise require a subtotal gastrectomy.

306. The answer is C. *(Schwartz, ed 5. pp 1198–1200.)* Regional enteritis may involve any segment of the GI tract from the esophagus to the rectum and often shows skip areas. The commonest area of involvement is the terminal ileum with minimal or no caecal involvement. The disease may also commonly involve both the small bowel and the right colon or present as jejunoileitis. The diarrhea in regional enteritis is of less frequency than that seen with ulcerative colitis and does not usually contain mucus, pus, or blood, although occult bleeding sufficient to produce anemia is a typical feature. Massive rectal bleeding is rare. The number of cases of adenocarcinoma of the small bowel associated with regional enteritis is small, but the association is probably significant. The 5-year survival is less than 10 percent. Although certain infectious agents such as enteroviruses, *Yersinia,* or *Campylobacter* have been linked to the acute variety of the disease, the cause of the typical chronic form is really not known. Viruses, immune deficiency, and genetic and toxic causes have all come under scrutiny as possible causes.

307. The answer is E. *(Schwartz, ed 5. pp 1209–1210.)* The malignant carcinoid syndrome is produced by excessive systemic levels of active biochemical substances secreted by a functioning carcinoid tumor. Serotonin, which is usually released by carcinoid metastases to the liver, is one of these substances. Although it was originally believed solely responsible for the syndrome, other active peptides and amines are now thought to be involved. The diagnosis of carcinoid syndrome is usually based on the presence of high urinary levels of 5-hydroxyindoleacetic acid (5-HIAA), which is a product of serotonin metabolism. In addition to the findings listed in the question, diarrhea, abdominal pain, malabsorption, and tricuspid valve disease are manifestations of the malignant carcinoid syndrome.

308. The answer is C. *(Schwartz, ed 5. pp 1525–1528.)* An indirect inguinal hernia leaves the abdominal cavity by entering the dilated internal inguinal ring and passing along the anteromedial aspect of the spermatic cord. The internal inguinal ring is an opening in the transversalis fascia for the passage of the spermatic cord; an indirect inguinal hernia, therefore, lies within the fibers of the cremaster muscle. Repair consists of removing the hernia sac and tightening the internal inguinal ring. A femoral hernia passes directly beneath the inguinal ligament at a point medial to the femoral vessels, and a *direct* inguinal hernia passes through a weakness in the floor of the inguinal canal medial to the inferior epigastric artery. Each is dependent on defects in Hesselbach's triangle of transversalis fascia and neither lies within the cremaster muscle fibers. Repair consists of reconstructing the floor of the inguinal canal. Spigelian hernias, which are rare, protrude through an anatomical defect that can occur along the lateral border of the rectus muscle at its junction with the linca semilunaris. An interparietal hernia is one in which the hernia sac, instead of protruding in the usual fashion, makes its way between the fascial layers of the abdominal wall. These unusual hernias may be preperitoneal (between the peritoneum and transversalis fascia), interstitial (between muscle layers), or superficial (between the external oblique aponeurosis and the skin).

309–310. The answers are: 309-D, 310-C. *(Schwartz, ed 5. pp 1393–1395.)* Gallstone ileus is due to erosion of a stone from the gallbladder into the gastrointestinal tract (most commonly into the duodenum). The stone becomes lodged in the small bowel—usually in the terminal ileum—and causes small bowel obstruction. Plain films of the abdomen demonstrating small bowel obstruction and air in the biliary tract are diagnostic of the condition. Treatment consists of enterotomy, removal of the stone, and cholecystectomy if it is technically safe. If there is significant right upper quadrant inflammation, enterotomy for stone extraction followed by an interval cholecystectomy is often a safer alternative.

311. The answer is A. *(Schwartz, ed 5. pp 1706–1707.)* Hirschsprung's disease—the congenital absence of ganglion cells in the rectum or rectosigmoid colon—is definitively diagnosed by rectal biopsy. The typical findings on barium enema, a distal narrow segment of bowel with markedly distended colon proximally, may not be seen early in life. Symptoms may go unrecognized in the newborn period with consequent development of malnutrition or enterocolitis. Initial treatment is colostomy decompression. Definitive repair is best delayed until nutritional status is adequate and the chronically distended bowel has returned to normal size. Unlike the situation with imperforate anus, which is associated with a high incidence of genitourinary tract anomalies and a 50 percent incidence of long-term fecal incontinence, in Hirschsprung's disease repair leads to satisfactory bowel function in most affected patients.

312. The answer is B. *(Schwartz, ed 5. pp 1694–1697.)* Esophageal atresia in association with tracheoesophageal fistula, the most common esophageal anomaly, involves a blind upper esophageal segment and a lower segment communicating with the trachea, usually at a point just above the bifurcation. Because the upper pouch is blind, regurgitation occurs but the affected infant is unable to belch. Coughing, copious mucus, and large amounts of air in the gastrointestinal tract are signs of communication between the lower esophageal segment and the trachea. There is a high association with other congenital anomalies, including cardiovascular disease (over 20 percent) and imperforate anus (12 percent). Over the past decade a variety of surgical techniques has evolved to improve the outlook for these infants; indeed, the most recent studies report that in over 80 percent of cases surgery has accomplished successful reconstitution of the intestinal tract.

313. The answer is D. *(Schwartz, ed 5. pp 1239, 1245, 1264–1268.)* Cancer of the colon in patients with chronic ulcerative colitis is ten times more frequent than in the general population. Duration of disease is very important; the risk of developing cancer in the first 10 years is low but thereafter rises about 4 percent per year. The average age of cancer development in patients with chronic ulcerative colitis is 37 years; idiopathic carcinoma of the colon, however, develops at an average age of 65 years. Crohn's colitis is currently felt to be a precancerous condition as well. The chance of development of carcinoma of the colon in patients with familial polyposis is essentially 100 percent. Treatment of the patient with familial polyposis generally consists of subtotal colectomy with ileoproctostomy and regular proctoscopic examination of the rectal stump. Villous adenomas have been demonstrated to contain malignant portions in about one-third of affected persons and invasive malignancy in another one-third of removed specimens. Anterior resection is performed for large lesions or those containing invasive carcinomas when the lesion is above the peritoneal reflection. Abdominoperineal resection is indicated for low-lying rectal villous adenomas when they have demonstrated invasive carcinomas. Transrectal excision with regular follow-up examinations is sufficient for lesions without invasive carcinomas. Peutz-Jeghers syndrome is characterized by intestinal polyposis and melanin spots of the oral mucosa. Unlike the adenomatous polyps seen in familial polyposis, the lesions in this condition are hamartomas, which have no malignant potential.

314. The answer is A. *(Schwartz, ed 5. pp 1712–1715.)* Omphalocele and gastroschisis result in evisceration of bowel and require emergency surgical treatment to effect immediate or staged reduction and abdominal wall closure. Patent urachal or omphalomesenteric ducts result from incomplete closure of embryonic connections from the bladder and ileum, respectively, to the abdominal wall. They are appropriately treated by excision of the tracts and closure of the bladder or ileum. In most children, umbilical hernias close spontaneously by the age of 4 and need not be repaired unless incarceration or marbled enlargement and distortion of the umbilicus occur.

315. The answer is C. *(Schwartz, ed 5. p 1494.)* Desmoid tumors are benign fibromas. They usually originate in the fascia of the anterior abdominal wall and can grow quite large in size. They may locally invade surrounding structures but have never been shown to metastasize. Some tumors will undergo malignant transformation to fibrosarcoma. The treatment of choice is wide local excision with reconstruction of the abdominal wall. Despite aggressive therapy, local recurrences are common and necessitate reexcision. No adjuvant therapy has proved to be of great benefit.

316. The answer is C. *(Schwartz, ed 5. p 1493.)* Hematomas of the rectus sheath are more common in women and present most often in the fifth decade. A history of trauma, sudden muscular exertion, or anticoagulation can usually be elicited. The pain is of sudden onset and is sharp in nature. The hematoma is most common in the right lower quadrant and irritation of the peritoneum leads to fever, leukocytosis, anorexia, and nausea. Preoperatively the diagnosis can be established with an ultrasound or CT scan showing a mass within the rectus sheath. Management is conservative unless symptoms are severe or bleeding persists, in which case surgical evacuation of the hematoma and ligation of bleeding vessels is required.

317. The answer is E. *(Schwartz, ed 5. pp 1347–1349.)* The liver is second only to regional lymph nodes as a site for metastatic spread of tumors. This is the most common form of hepatic malignancy, with the relative ratio of secondary to primary neoplasms being about 20:1. About 25 to 50 percent of all patients dying of cancer have hepatic metastases and about 50 percent of all patients with gastrointestinal tumors have hepatic metastases at autopsy. The incidence of hepatoma or primary hepatocellular carcinoma is relatively rare in populations from North America and Western Europe, although it is common in certain parts of Africa where primary liver cancer represents 17 to 53 percent of all cancers. Angiosarcoma rarely occurs in the liver, though when it does it has been associated with exposure to vinyl chloride. Hamartomas and hemangiomas are fairly common benign neoplasms of the liver.

318. The answer is E. *(Schwartz, ed 5. pp 1708–1718.)* Congenital anorectal anomalies are frequently associated with other congenital anomalies including heart disease, esophageal atresia, abnormalities of the lumbosacral spine, double urinary collecting systems, hydronephrosis, and communication between the rectum and the urinary tract, vagina, or perineum. Congenital anorectal anomalies are not as common as congenital megacolon (Hirschsprung's disease), and their cause is unknown. They occur in approximately 1 in 2000 live births. Depending on the type of anomaly, a variety of surgical procedures has been devised to treat the problem. However, even when anatomic integrity is established, the prognosis for effective toilet training is poor. In 50 percent of cases continence is never achieved. Corneal opacities have no significant association with congenital anorectal anomalies.

319. The answer is B. *(Schwartz, ed 5. pp 1418–1419.)* Although the actual pathogenesis of acute pancreatitis is unknown, the condition most commonly occurs in association with either cholelithiasis or alcoholism. Other disorders associated with acute pancreatitis (including peptic ulcer, trauma, surgery, hyperlipoproteinemia, hypercalcemia, hereditary factors, infections, and administration of certain drugs) are so diverse that it is difficult to postulate a single responsible pathophysiologic mechanism. Hypothyroidism has not been noted to be associated with pancreatitis.

320. The answer is A. *(Schwartz, ed 5. p 1357.)* Massive hematemesis in children is almost always due to variceal bleeding. The varices usually result from extrahepatic portal vein obstruction consequent to bacterial infection transmitted via a patent umbilical vein during infancy. In spite of this common cause, a history of neonatal omphalitis is infrequently obtainable. Bleeding can be massive but is usually self-limited and esophageal tamponade or vasopressin is usually not necessary. Elective portal-systemic decompression is recommended for recurrent bleeding episodes.

321. The answer is C (2, 4). *(Schwartz, ed 5. pp 1704–1705.)* Intussusception is the result of invagination of a segment of bowel into distal bowel lumen. The most common type is ileocolic, typically presenting a coiled spring appearance on barium enema. Ileoileal and colocolic intussusceptions occur less commonly and are not easily diagnosed on barium enema. If bloody mucus, peritonitis, or systemic toxicity have not developed, hydrostatic reduction by barium enema is the appropriate initial treatment. Most patients are successfully managed this way and do not require surgical intervention. Immediate treatment should be instituted to avert the danger of bowel infarction. Recurrence is surprisingly uncommon after either surgical or nonsurgical treatment.

322. The answer is A (1, 2, 3). *(Sabiston, ed 13. pp 821–822.)* Acute stress ulceration of the gastroduodenal mucosae occurs commonly in patients who are in an intensive care unit. These ulcers have been called Cushing's ulcers when seen in patients with head trauma and have been referred to as Curling's ulcers in patients with major burns. The exact mechanism of formation is not well understood but does seem to include the presence of acid (excess acid is not required), ischemia of the mucosa, and a breakdown of the mucosal barrier. Sepsis seems to be the most common cause. Prophylaxis with antacids (gastric pH greater than 3.5) will significantly reduce the incidence of these potentially life-threatening lesions.

323. The answer is C (2, 4). *(Brooks, pp 263–279.)* The vast majority of pancreatic carcinomas are located in the head of the gland. Patients may present with painless jaundice by virtue of the carcinoma's obstruction of the intrapancreatic portion of the common bile duct. It is in this group of patients that resection is even possible—although most will be unresectable. Tumors in the body or tail of the gland are universally unresectable. The cause of pancreatic cancer is not known. There is a very strong association with diabetes mellitus but the nature of this relationship is not known. Prognosis is uniformly dismal whether resection is done or not and only an anecdotal survivor will be alive at 5-year follow-up.

324. The answer is D (4). *(Sabiston, ed 13. pp 949–952, 976.)* Carcinoid tumors arise from the neuroectoderm and are a type of apudoma. The most common site of carcinoid tumors is the small bowel. The appendix is a rare site of carcinoids, but the location is associated with a good prognosis. Carcinoid syndrome, which is characterized by flushing, diarrhea, and cardiac valvular disease, occurs in a small percentage of patients with carcinoid tumors and can be seen with appendiceal carcinoids. The appropriate therapy for a small carcinoid (less than 2 cm) of the appendix is simple appendectomy.

325. The answer is D (4). *(Sabiston, ed 13. p 995.)* The sigmoid colon, with its large redundant loop on a narrow-based mesentery, is prone to volvulus. There is commonly a long history of constipation and laxative use. The passage of a lubricated rectal tube through a rigid proctoscope is often sufficient to decompress the sigmoid colon and permit the volvulus to untwist. Colonoscopic decompression has also been used with success. Should these maneuvers fail to decompress the volvulus or there are signs of gangrene, an emergency sigmoid colectomy should be performed. Otherwise the rectal tube is left in place, the bowel prepared, and colonoscopy performed to rule out coexistent malignancies. More than 50 percent of these patients will experience a recurrence if untreated. The preferred management is elective resection of the sigmoid colon with primary anastomosis.

326. The answer is E (all). *(Schwartz, ed 5. pp 1392–1393.)* The management of retained stones of the common bile duct has progressed considerably in recent years. Nonoperative therapy has become the most common route of management with basket retrieval via the T-tube tract successful in 96 percent of cases. If no T tube is in place, papillotomy via endoscopic retrograde cholangiopancreatography (ERCP) will allow stone passage in about 86 percent of cases. Chemical dissolution is less attractive because of the prolonged course of treatment, but it is also successful greater than 50 percent of the time. Surgical intervention is reserved for cases in which other techniques have failed.

327. The answer is A (1, 2, 3). *(Sabiston, ed 13. pp 1189–1192.)* Pancreatic pseudocysts can develop in the setting of acute and chronic pancreatitis. They are cystic collections that do not have an epithelial lining. Most pseudocysts will spontaneously resolve. Therapy should not be considered for 6 weeks to allow for the possibility of spontaneous resolution as well as to allow for maturation of the cyst wall if the cyst persists. Complications of pseudocysts include gastric outlet and extrahepatic biliary obstructions as well as spontaneous rupture and hemorrhage. Pseudocysts can be excised, externally drained, or internally drained into the gastrointestinal tract (most commonly the stomach or a Roux en Y limb of jejunum).

328. The answer is C (2, 4). *(Sabiston, ed 13. pp 1240–1246.)* Direct inguinal hernias occur medial to the inferior epigastric vessels and are best repaired by reapproximating the transversalis fascia to Cooper's ligament and thus reconstructing the floor of the inguinal canal. The hernia sac is opened and ligated routinely during indirect hernia repair but not during direct hernia repair. The most common inguinal hernia in women is an indirect hernia.

329. The answer is D (4). *(Way, ed 7. p 499.)* A radionuclide excretion scan is a useful diagnostic study in patients suspected of having acute cholecystitis. A variety of radionuclide materials can be used (HIDA is one example); they are given intravenously, thereby eliminating the need for GI absorption. The test does not actually demonstrate gallstones but rather it will show obstruction of the cystic duct in the setting of acute cholecystitis. It can be done in patients with dye allergy and in patients with bilirubins as high as 15 to 20 mg%. A small number of false positives can be seen in patients with advanced chronic gallbladder inflammation, and in patients with other unrelated intraabdominal pathology. The scan shown is a good example of a scan that documents obstruction of the cystic duct.

330. The answer is B (1, 3). *(Schwartz, ed 5. pp 1286–1287.)* Chemotherapeutic agents have been of little benefit in treating patients with colorectal carcinomas whether used as an adjuvant or for palliation of metastatic disease. Radiotherapy is usually ineffective because colorectal carcinomas are not radiosensitive tumors and the gastrointestinal tract does not tolerate radiation very well.

331. The answer is A (1, 2, 3). *(Schwartz, ed 5. p 1089.)* Pitressin decreases portal vein pressure and P_{O_2}. It also decreases cardiac output and gastric mucosal perfusion, while increasing peripheral blood pressure, by constricting splanchnic vessels. There is no evidence that selective Pitressin is more effective than peripheral Pitressin in controlling gastrointestinal hemorrhage.

332. The answer is C (2, 4). *(Schwartz, ed 5. p 1391.)* Although somewhat controversial, cholecystectomy should generally be performed in the good-risk asymptomatic patient. Symptoms will ultimately develop in 50 percent of patients, with serious complications including obstruction of the common duct in as many as 20 percent. The operative mortality increases from less than 1 percent for elective surgery to 5 percent in patients with acute cholecystitis. Although the incidence of carcinoma in patients with symptomatic cholelithiasis averages 4.5 percent, the incidence in patients with asymptomatic stones is probably less than 1 percent. There is no recognized relation between gallstones and hepatic cirrhosis.

333. The answer is C (2, 4). *(Schwartz, ed 5. p 1260.)* Cecal diverticula must be differentiated from the more common variety of diverticula that are usually found in the left colon. Cecal diverticula are thought to be a congenital entity. The cecal diverticulum is often solitary and involves all layers of the bowel wall; therefore, cecal diverticula are true diverticula. Diverticula elsewhere in the colon are almost always multiple and are thought to be an acquired disorder. These acquired diverticula are really herniations of mucosa through weakened areas of the muscularis propria of the colon wall. The preoperative diagnosis in the case of cecal diverticulitis is "acute appendicitis" about 80 percent of the time. If there is extensive inflammation involving much of the cecum, an ileocolectomy is indicated. If the inflammation is well localized to the area of diverticulum, a simple diverticulectomy with closure of the defect is the procedure of choice. To avoid diagnostic confusion in the future, the appendix should be removed whenever an incision is made in the right lower quadrant, unless operatively contraindicated.

334. The answer is C (2, 4). *(Schwartz, ed 5. pp 1178–1179.)* Most gastric polyps are not true neoplasms but are inflammatory in nature. Adenomatous gastric polyps, as is the case with adenomatous colonic polyps, have the potential to undergo malignant transformation. All polyps found in the stomach should be biopsied endoscopically and those found to be adenomatous should be removed using standard endoscopic polypectomy techniques. Polyps found to contain invasive malignancy should be managed by gastric resection. Although the polyps are usually unnoticed by the patient, they may produce obstructive symptoms if they prolapse through the pylorus. Patients with pernicious anemia (atrophic gastritis) need to be watched for the development of neoplastic gastric polyps.

335. The answer is D (4). *(Schwartz, ed 5. p 1421.)* Acute peritonitis generally mandates celiotomy. An important exception is the peritonitis resulting from pancreatitis, which is usually treated by conservative measures because operative intervention increases mortality (acute hemorrhagic pancreatitis is often the exception). Whatever the degree of hypocalcemia associated with pancreatitis, it is treated medically. Pancreatic pseudocysts, which may be associated with either chronic or acute pancreatitis, are often symptomatic or lead to complications such as abscess formation. These may resolve spontaneously or be managed by percutaneous drainage. In some cases, surgical decompression is necessary. For patients with gallstone pancreatitis, removal of common duct stones surgically or endoscopically can reduce morbidity and mortality.

336. The answer is A (1, 2, 3). *(Schwartz, ed 5. p 1421.)* Acute pancreatitis is usually treated by withholding administration of all fluids and foods by mouth, placing a nasogastric tube for intermittent suction, and administering parenteral analgesics (meperidine is preferred) and fluids. Adjuncts to this therapy may include administration of anticholinergic agents, calcium gluconate, and antacids. In hemorrhagic pancreatitis, more aggressive therapy occasionally may be required, including blood transfusions and surgery. Although some workers still advocate the use of antibiotics, most now recommend their use only for specific indications in unusual cases. Use of the nasogastric tube is generally recommended, although several controlled studies cast doubt regarding its benefit, particularly in the presence of significant patient discomfort. Steroids are not recommended as they may cause pancreatitis.

337. The answer is A (1, 2, 3). *(Schwartz, ed 5. p 1532.)* Under certain circumstances, the usual approach to abdominal wall hernias, surgical repair, may not be warranted. Congenital umbilical hernias usually resolve spontaneously and surgery is not indicated before the age of 4 in the absence of complications. Elderly high-risk surgical patients with asymptomatic inguinal hernias also may be reasonably managed expectantly. Although trusses are generally not successful, the patient with a large ventral hernia, where surgical repair may be difficult, can be successfully managed nonoperatively with a properly fitted corset and close follow-up. Injection of sclerosing solutions into tissues around a hernia is not an effective treatment option.

338. The answer is B (1, 3). *(Schwartz, ed 5. pp 1335–1337.)* The most common organism in liver abscesses is *E. coli* (50 percent). Amebic abscess usually involves the right lobe and has a high male predominance. The highest percentage of cases of pyogenic liver abscess occurs in the sixth and seventh decades of life and usually results from biliary infection, hematogenous spread via the portal vein, or septicemia. Blood cultures are diagnostic in only about 50 percent of cases. Gram-negative and anaerobic (bacteroides) organisms are increasing in frequency as causes of pyogenic hepatic abscess. Infection with *Entamoeba histolytica* is much more common than many suspect (>10 percent of the U.S. population). Amebas reach the liver via portal venous blood from an area of bowel ulceration, thereafter producing single or multiple abscess cavities containing "anchovy paste" purulence. Bacterial superinfection and rupture are serious complications of amebic abscess. Therapy consists of metronidazole, which acts on both intestinal and hepatic amebas, followed by aspiration or surgical drainage. Although tuberculosis peritonitis still occasionally occurs in this country, tuberculous hepatic abscesses are very rare.

339. The answer is A (1, 2, 3). *(Schwartz, ed 5. pp 1132–1133.)* Pharyngoesophageal diverticulum is an acquired abnormality usually seen in patients over 50 years of age. Dysphagia is common and is the usual presenting symptom. The diagnosis is established by barium swallow. Treatment is surgical—diverticulectomy or suspension of the diverticulum is usually recommended. Because the diverticulum is located above the superior esophageal sphincter, no mechanism exists to prevent aspiration of the contents of the diverticulum. Pulmonary complications are common.

340–341. The answers are: 340-A (1, 2, 3), 341-B (1, 3). *(Starker, pp 261–264.)* With proper management the majority of enterocutaneous fistulas can be expected to close spontaneously. This management must include gaining control of the fistula by obtaining adequate drainage of the abscess cavity and preventing ongoing local sepsis or generalized sepsis. The management of fluid and electrolyte losses is crucial, especially in high-output proximal fistulas. The corrosive action of the enteric contents on the skin of the abdominal wall must be prevented by use of sump drains or ostomy equipment. Proximal diversion is not necessary if the fistula can be controlled with the previously mentioned measures. Over the next 4 to 6 weeks the fistula can be expected to close if adequate nutrition is supplied. The enteral route is the preferred route. If the fistula is a proximal, high-output one, it may be difficult to provide enough nutrition enterally and the fistula will not heal, not because of the high volume but because of the failure to deliver nutrients. In this case parenteral nutrition is indicated. Distal obstruction, foreign bodies, cancer, epithelialization of the tract, and ongoing infection all tend to prevent spontaneous closure of a fistula.

342. The answer is E (all). *(Schwartz, ed 5. p 1434.)* The metabolic consequences of total pancreatectomy are manifold. They include weight loss, malabsorption attended by hypocalcemia and hypophosphatemia, diabetes mellitus, diarrhea, and both iron deficiency and pernicious anemia. In theory, total pancreatectomy should provide good surgical treatment for pancreatic carcinoma; in reality, the severe metabolic problems that result from total removal of the pancreas make partial pancreaticoduodenectomy a frequently preferred treatment for most cases of pancreatic carcinoma that are resectable. Because of the frequently multicentric nature of pancreatic cancers, however, some surgeons would rather perform a total pancreatectomy and accept the more complicated postoperative metabolic management entailed by the loss of pancreatic endocrine function.

343. The answer is A (1, 2, 3). *(Schwartz, ed 5. p 1399.)* Cholangitis is suggested by the presence of Charcot's triad: fever, jaundice, and right upper quadrant pain. These symptoms are usually caused by choledocholithiasis but they can also occur in association with obstructing neoplasms and choledochal cysts. Therapy is aimed at decompression of the common bile duct. This is usually best accomplished by surgical placement of a T tube into the duct. Percutaneous transhepatic catheter drainage is an acceptable alternative in select patients. This procedure often can provide effective decompression during the acute septic phase of the disease. Cholecystostomy will be effective only if there is free flow of bile into the gallbladder via the cystic duct and in general should not be depended on to secure drainage of the common bile duct.

344. The answer is E (all). *(Schwartz, ed 5. pp 1239–1241.)* Ulcerative colitis is an inflammatory disease of the colon causing crampy abdominal pain, diarrhea, and blood per rectum. In addition, this disorder exhibits several extracolonic manifestations, including arthritis, erythema nodosum, pyoderma gangrenosum, chronic active hepatitis, sclerosing cholangitis, and ocular lesions. Colonic complications of chronic ulcerative colitis include carcinoma of the colon, toxic megacolon, and perforation. Seventy-five to eighty percent of patients with the disease can be managed medically; in the remaining patients, total proctocolectomy and ileostomy is currently the procedure of choice.

345. The answer is A (1, 2, 3). *(Schwartz, ed 5. pp 1391–1392.)* Various criteria provide indications for exploration of the common bile duct; these include palpable stones in the common bile duct, dilatation of the duct (the normal diameter is less than 1 cm), the history or presence of jaundice, pancreatitis, and numerous small calculi in the gallbladder in the presence of a relatively large cystic duct. In an effort to avoid negative exploration of the duct, routine operative cholangiograms have been advocated by some authors. With this technique, the incidence of explorations of the common duct in conjunction with cholecystectomy has been reduced from 65 to 29 percent in one series, whereas the incidence of positive explorations was increased from 23 to 66 percent. New techniques involving the use of intraoperative choledochoscopes may further reduce the frequency of negative explorations of the duct.

346. The answer is A (1, 2, 3). *(Sabiston, ed 13. pp 756–758. Schwartz, ed 5. p 1122.)* Paraesophageal hernia results from a diaphragmatic defect. The stomach herniates into the chest, a situation that can lead to strangulation, hemorrhage, or obstruction. Because of the potential for such problems, surgical repair is indicated even in an affected patient who is asymptomatic. Paraesophageal hernia contrasts with the more common sliding esophageal hiatal hernia, in which obstruction occurs only after a prolonged period of untreated esophagitis and in which strangulation would not be expected to develop. Reflux esophagitis is seen in some patients with hiatal hernia, but not with paraesophageal hernia.

347. The answer is E (all). *(Schwartz, ed 5. p 1254.)* Diverticulosis affects about ten million people in the United States and often is asymptomatic. Diverticula do not cause symptoms unless they are complicated by bleeding or inflammation. While the pathogenesis is not completely understood, all the factors listed in the question are believed to contribute to the development of diverticulosis. Additionally, patients who have the irritable bowel syndrome are now thought to be prone to acquire this condition. A high-bulk diet is considered preventive.

348. The answer is A (1, 2, 3). *(Schwartz, ed 5. pp 1170–1173.)* Although subtotal (70 percent) gastrectomy at one time was commonly performed for persons with peptic ulcer disease (PUD), fewer and fewer surgeons are using this procedure for elective treatment. Most of them prefer vagotomy with some form of drainage procedure—either pyloroplasty, gastrojejunostomy, or antrectomy. The differences among these procedures have to do with the relative incidences of recurrent ulceration and operative morbidity and mortality. Vagotomy and antrectomy have the lowest ulcer recurrence rates (1 to 2 percent in most series), but are associated with a somewhat higher operative mortality (1.5 to 3 percent) when compared with vagotomy and pyloroplasty or gastrojejunostomy, which carry a recurrence of 5 to 7 percent with operative mortality of less than 1 percent. Proximal or parietal cell vagotomy has the advantage of not requiring drainage and thereby avoiding such consequences as gastrointestinal dysfunction and the dumping syndrome. Unfortunately, although the mortality associated with this procedure is very low (less than 1 percent), parietal cell vagotomy is of too recent advent to permit accurate comparison of recurrence rates. Late recurrence rates may be as high as 8 to 10 percent. Gastroenterostomy alone, which began as a means for treating outlet obstruction secondary to PUD, should never be performed for PUD because the antral alkalinization by pancreatic and biliary secretions leads to increased gastrin secretions and frequent ulcer diathesis. Marginal ulcers will develop in many patients treated this way.

349. The answer is B (1, 3). *(Schwartz, ed 5. pp 1423–1424.)* Although the surgical treatment of chronic abdominal pain caused by chronic alcoholic pancreatitis is not entirely satisfactory, some affected patients with a dilated pancreatic duct (>8 mm) can be helped by anastomosis of the distal pancreatic duct to the jejunum. The rationale for this approach is based on the observation that the diseased pancreatic duct frequently is strictured in the head of the organ and drainage is ineffective. Communication between the duct and a segment of jejunum can be accomplished by a pancreaticojejunostomy of the type described by Puestow. Distal pancreaticojejunostomy does not afford adequate drainage of the pancreatic duct. When the pancreas is diffusely involved with chronic disease and the pancreatic duct is not strictured, a 95 percent distal pancreatectomy may offer relief from pain, but at the cost of incurring a high incidence of diabetes and exocrine pancreatic insufficiency. Sympathectomy has been attempted but there is no evidence that it is helpful in relieving the pain of chronic pancreatitis.

350. The answer is D (4). *(Schwartz, ed 5. p 1212.)* Meckel's diverticulum is found on the antimesenteric border of the ileum within the first 3 feet of the ileocecal valve. It may contain gastric mucosa and peptic ulceration may lead to bleeding. However, the most common complication in affected adults is obstruction. This may result from volvulus of a portion of intestine around a band that can sometimes be seen extending from the tip of the diverticulum to the umbilicus or abdominal wall. Obstruction may be due to intussusception, with the diverticulum being the lead point.

351. The answer is B (1, 3). *(Schwartz, ed 5. pp 1257–1258.)* The most likely diagnosis in this patient is perforated diverticulitis or carcinoma. The chest film shows air beneath the right hemidiaphragm, indicating a free perforation. Although this patient does not yet show any other signs of generalized peritonitis, immediate exploration of the abdomen is indicated. This elderly woman needs to receive large volumes of intravenous fluid over a short period of time in preparation for surgery. Moreover, she is at high risk for septic shock. A central venous catheter and indwelling Foley catheter should be inserted immediately. Colonoscopy introduces large amounts of air into the colon, which might worsen the fecal spillage. If there were no signs of free perforation, an ultrasound examination would be useful to diagnose abscess, since an abscess (resulting from localized perforation) is not likely to respond to antibiotics alone. Intestinal ischemia from thrombosis or embolus is a life-threatening condition that requires immediate operation but can be difficult to diagnose. Elderly patients in atrial fibrillation are particularly at risk.

352–356. The answers are: 352-C, 353-A, 354-B, 355-B, 356-D. *(Sabiston, ed 13. pp 1177–1188.)* Inflammation of the pancreas presents clinically as a spectrum of disease. Acute pancreatitis is commonly seen in association with alcohol use and gallstones. The histopathology may range from minimal edema to hemorrhagic necrosis (both are always reversible). Chronic pancreatitis is felt to be caused by chronic alcohol abuse but not generally by gallstones. Fibrosis and calcification of the gland is seen with chronic pancreatitis and these changes are irreversible. Patients with either acute or chronic pancreatitis are not at higher risk for the development of pancreatic cancer compared with the general population. Both may lead to the formation of pseudocysts. ERCP is used frequently in the evaluation of patients with chronic pancreatitis but is contraindicated in patients with active acute pancreatitis.

357–361. The answers are: 357-B, 358-C, 359-C, 360-B, 361-D. *(Way, ed 8. pp 616–623.)* Ulcerative colitis and Crohn's colitis are each forms of inflammatory bowel disease. Ulcerative colitis is a chronic inflammatory disease limited to the colonic mucosa. The rectum is almost always involved and the colon may be involved as well in a continuous distribution. Ulcerative colitis is a major risk factor for the development of carcinoma of the colon and approximately 5 percent of patients will develop a carcinoma after 10 years of ulcerative colitis. Crohn's colitis is a transmural inflammatory disease of the colon in which chronic inflammation (with granuloma formation) is seen in all layers of the colon. It frequently spares the rectum (50 percent of cases) and involves the remainder of the colon segmentally with skip areas. Crohn's colitis is also felt to be a precancerous lesion. Colonoscopy is commonly performed in both. Toxic megacolon may complicate either ulcerative colitis or Crohn's colitis. Sclerosing cholangitis is associated with both; however, perianal fistulas are generally seen only with Crohn's colitis.

362–365. The answers are: 362-D, 363-A, 364-B, 365-E. *(Schwartz, ed 5. pp 271, 1430, 1447. Sabiston, ed 13. pp 1139, 1180.)* Patients with splenic rupture may relate a history of pain at the tip of the left shoulder (Kehr's sign), which is caused by the irritation of the left hemidiaphragm by blood. This pain might only occur when the patient is in a supine or head-down position. It occurs in less than half of patients with splenic rupture.

In a patient with acute cholecystitis deep inspiration with the examiner's hand on the right upper quadrant will cause the gallbladder to move caudad and strike the parietal peritoneum causing pain (Murphy's sign).

Acute pancreatitis, if severe and hemorrhagic, may result in the tracking of blood through the tissue planes of the retroperitoneal space. Discoloration of the skin of the flanks (Grey Turner's sign) and of the periumbilical region (Cullen's sign) may occur.

Patients with obstructive jaundice secondary to pancreatic cancer will often present with a dilated, palpable gallbladder (Courvoisier's sign). This is not always present because the gallbladder may be fibrotic and nondistensible owing to chronic inflammation from gallstones or the cystic duct may be occluded by the tumor.

366–370. The answers are: 366-A, 367-C, 368-B, 369-E, 370-D. *(Schwartz, ed 5. pp 1526–1530.)* The indirect inguinal hernia is commonly seen in young children and is easily repaired by simple ligation of the sac. If not repaired in childhood, the internal inguinal ring tends to widen as the person matures and a more extensive repair is necessary to close the internal ring and prevent recurrence.

A direct inguinal hernia is due to a weakness in the floor of Hesselbach's triangle, the anatomic area bounded by the inferior epigastric artery, inguinal ligament, and lateral margin of the rectus sheath. Because of the inherent tissue weakness, recurrence is more likely following repair of this type of hernia than other types of groin hernias.

Umbilical hernias are common in infants, but often will close by 5 years of age and therefore do not require repair unless they cause symptoms or become complicated by incarceration. Repair is indicated, however, when these hernias are found later in life, especially in cirrhotic patients with ascites, or in women with enlarged fascial defects following pregnancy.

Femoral hernias may be difficult to diagnose because of their location deep to the inguinal ligament, a difficulty that may be particularly troublesome in the obese patient. These hernias should be sought in any patient who presents with bowel obstruction.

A sliding hernia is one in which one wall of the sac (commonly posterior) is made up of a viscus. Whenever a hernia sac is opened, this possibility must be kept in mind in order to avoid injury to bowel or other sliding component.

An omphalocele represents a more severe congenital variant of the umbilical hernia. A fascial defect is present but, in addition, the bowel is covered only by peritoneum. As the peritoneal surface dries out in the early days of life, serious bowel complications can occur.

371–374. The answers are: 371-D, 372-D, 373-C, 374-E. *(Schwartz, ed 5. pp 1119–1124.)* Paraesophageal hernias, generally thought to be acquired, involve herniation of any portion or all of the stomach into the thoracic cavity via the esophageal hiatus. These hernias are usually repaired electively because of a high incidence of complications. In these dangerous hernias, the cardioesophageal junction is in its normal position below the diaphragm.

Diaphragmatic ruptures usually affect adults and result from blunt trauma to the abdomen. Unless such ruptures are repaired, the negative intrathoracic pressure associated with each respiratory effort tends to suck the abdominal contents into the chest with consequent loss of necessary space for lung expansion and substantial risk of damage to the intrathoracic bowel.

Sliding hiatal hernias, the most frequent type of hernia found in adults, generally are acquired. The significance of this type of hernia rests in its association with gastroesophageal reflux, a condition that may lead to reflux esophagitis. Because sliding hiatal hernias frequently do not exhibit significant gastroesophageal reflux, it is likely that other factors may be more important in the pathophysiology of that disorder.

The foramen of Bochdalek hernia is a congenital hernia of the posterolateral aspect of the diaphragm, in which abdominal viscera enter the thorax and cause acute respiratory distress in infants. This hernia requires emergency repair.

The foramen of Morgagni hernia, although also congenital, is not usually detected until adulthood. It is usually an incidental finding on chest x-ray, appearing as a low anterior mediastinal mass. However, on rare occasions it can produce acute respiratory distress in infants.

Cardiothoracic Problems

DIRECTIONS: Each question below contains five suggested responses. Select the **one best** response to each question.

375. Cardiac transplant rejection is monitored by

(A) periodic endomyocardial biopsy
(B) cardiac output
(C) blood pressure
(D) WBC and platelet count
(E) decreased ECG voltage

Questions 376–377

376. A noncyanotic 2-day-old child has a systolic murmur along the left sternal border; the examination is otherwise normal. Chest x-ray and electrocardiogram are normal. These findings are most closely associated with which of the following congenital cardiac anomalies?

(A) Tetralogy of Fallot
(B) Ventricular septal defect
(C) Tricuspid atresia
(D) Transposition of the great vessels
(E) Patent ductus arteriosus

377. A 3-year-old child with congenital cyanosis most probably is suffering from

(A) tetralogy of Fallot
(B) ventricular septal defect
(C) tricuspid atresia
(D) transposition of the great vessels
(E) patent ductus arteriosus

378. The poorest prognosis of aortic stenosis is associated with which of the following signs or symptoms?

(A) Angina pectoris
(B) Congestive failure
(C) Palpitation
(D) Exertional dyspnea
(E) Syncope

379. A 52-year-old white woman undergoing routine physical examination has the chest x-ray shown below. The lesion present was not seen on x-rays taken 6 years previously. The patient, who has a 20-year history of smoking, is asymptomatic. Physical examination, bronchoscopy, and sputum cytology disclose no significant findings. At the time of operation a firm lesion is removed. It is sectioned in the operating room, revealing tissue that looks like cartilage and smooth muscle along with epithelial elements. The tumor is most probably

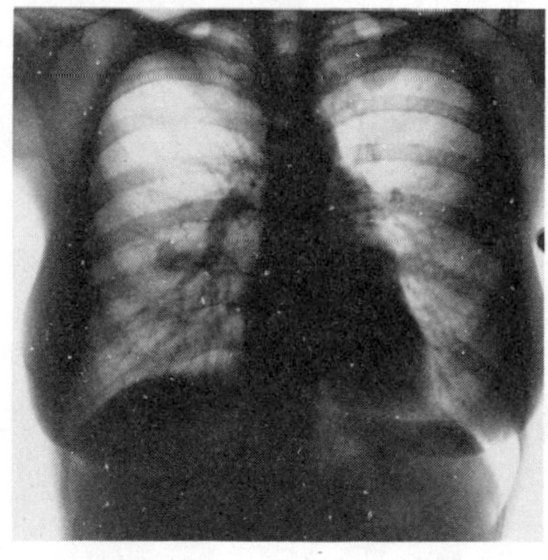

(A) a chondroma
(B) a teratoma
(C) a hamartoma
(D) a chondrosarcoma
(E) an osteochondroma

380. A 4-year-old boy is seen 1 hour after ingestion of a lye drain cleaner. No oropharyngeal burns are noted, but his voice is hoarse. Chest x-ray is normal. Of the following, which is the most appropriate therapy?

(A) Immediate esophagoscopy
(B) Parenteral steroids and antibiotics
(C) Administration of an oral neutralizing agent
(D) Induction of vomiting
(E) Rapid administration of a quart of water to clear remaining lye from the esophagus and dilute material in stomach

381. A 35-year-old woman, who has signs and symptoms of mitral stenosis, is found to have a 3-cm tumor in the left atrium. This mass is most likely to be

(A) metastatic carcinoma
(B) malignant lymphoma
(C) hemangioma
(D) rhabdomyoma
(E) myxoma

382. Mediastinal emphysema is likely to have all the following physical manifestations EXCEPT

(A) cyanosis
(B) acute left heart failure
(C) systolic crunch
(D) substernal pain
(E) sore throat

383. An 8-year-old boy is brought to a physician because of palpitation, fatigue, and dyspnea. On examination a continuous machinery murmer is heard best in the second left intercostal space and is widely transmitted over the precordium. The most likely diagnosis is

(A) ventricular septal defect
(B) atrial septal defect
(C) congenital aortic stenosis
(D) patent ductus arteriosus
(E) coarctation of the aorta

384. Which of the following treatments is indicated for a patient who has the condition shown in the x-ray below?

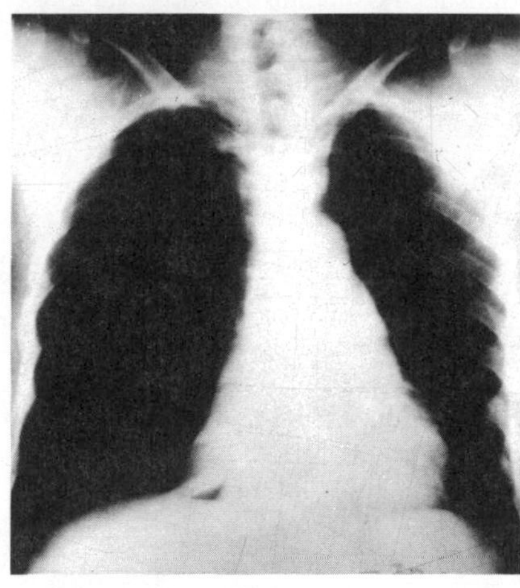

(A) Bed rest and observation
(B) Positive-pressure ventilation
(C) Bronchoscopy
(D) Insertion of a chest tube
(E) Thoracotomy for pleurodesis

Questions 385–386

A 60-year-old man complains of chest pain suggestive of angina. Physical examination reveals a ''diamond-shaped'' systolic murmur with no evidence of congestive heart failure. Cardiac catheterization reveals the coronary arteries to be relatively free of demonstrable disease.

385. In the patient presented, the lesion defined by catheterization is most likely to be

(A) tricuspid insufficiency
(B) mitral insufficiency
(C) mitral stenosis
(D) aortic stenosis
(E) acquired ventricular septal defect

386. Correct management of the patient described above would involve

(A) digoxin administration
(B) coronary vasodilator administration
(C) valve replacement
(D) an exercise program
(E) none of the above

387. Mitral stenosis is associated with all the following conditions EXCEPT

(A) hemoptysis
(B) arterial emboli
(C) low left atrial pressures
(D) atrial fibrillation
(E) tricuspid insufficiency

388. The superior vena cava syndrome is most frequently seen in association with

(A) histoplasmosis (sclerosing mediastinitis)
(B) substernal thyroid
(C) thoracic aortic aneurysm
(D) constrictive pericarditis
(E) bronchogenic carcinoma

389. A previously healthy 20-year-old man is admitted to a hospital with acute onset of left sided chest pain. The electrocardiographic findings are normal but chest x-ray shows a 40 percent left pneumothorax. Treatment consists of which of the following procedures?

(A) Observation
(B) Barium swallow
(C) Thoracotomy
(D) Tube thoracostomy
(E) Thoracostomy and intubation

390. A 45-year-old woman was found at the wheel of her car after a high-speed motor vehicle accident. On arrival in the emergency room, she is in severe respiratory distress, with a systolic blood pressure of 90 mmHg. Examination reveals crepitus and paradoxical movement of a large segment of the right chest. A right sided chest tube is placed without improvement in her respiratory status and the decision is made to intubate. She is now thrashing around in agitation. All the following are indicated EXCEPT

(A) cricoid pressure (Sellick maneuver)
(B) a left sided chest tube
(C) administration of 2 mg/kg ketamine intravenously for sedation
(D) administration of 3 mg/kg of curare for muscle relaxation
(E) axial traction applied to the head

391. Pleural mesotheliomas have been associated with all the following EXCEPT

(A) a history of asbestos exposure
(B) a history of thoracic trauma
(C) pulmonary osteoarthropathy
(D) cigarette smoking
(E) hypoglycemia

392. Rupture of the thoracic aorta associated with closed chest trauma most commonly occurs

(A) in the ascending aorta
(B) in the transverse aorta proximal to the left subclavian artery
(C) in the proximal descending aorta
(D) with equal distribution throughout the aorta
(E) at the level of the diaphragm

393. An 89-year-old man has lost 30 pounds over the past 2 years. He reports that food frequently sticks when he swallows. He also complains of a chronic cough. Pulmonary function tests show a vital capacity of 60 percent of expected, and forced expiratory volume is 50 percent of predicted. Barium swallow is shown below. Which of the following statements is true?

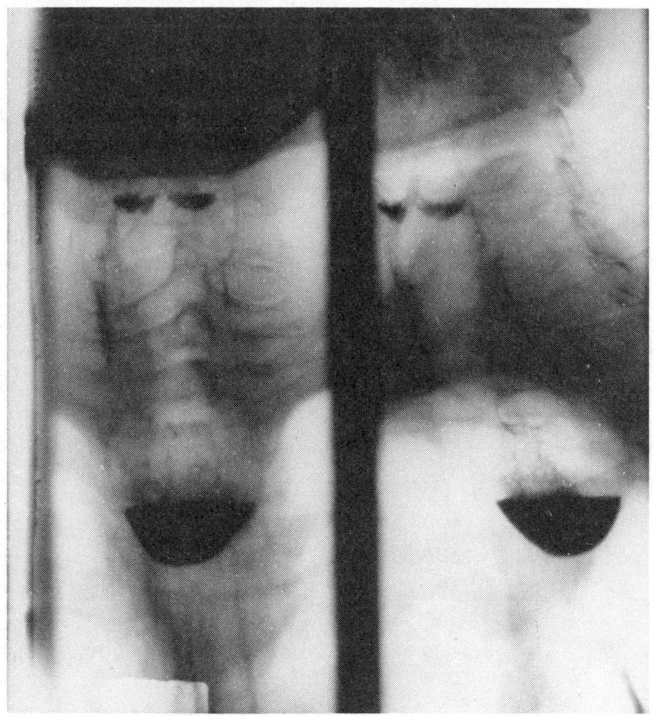

(A) Radiation therapy and stenting can be expected to produce the same long-term survival as would surgery
(B) Esophagoscopy and biopsy should be performed to confirm the x-ray findings
(C) This patient is atypical in that the lesion usually appears in the second or third decade of life
(D) The patient should be treated with antituberculous medications before any surgical intervention is considered
(E) The carotid bifurcation lies adjacent to the lesion

Questions 394–395

Several days following esophagectomy a patient complains of dyspnea and chest tightness. A large pleural effusion is noted on chest radiograph and thoracentesis yields milky fluid consistent with chyle.

394. Initial management of this patient consists of which of the following procedures?

(A) Immediate operation to repair the thoracic duct
(B) Immediate operation to ligate the thoracic duct
(C) Observation and low-fat diet
(D) Tube thoracostomy and low-fat diet
(E) Observation and antibiotics

395. Two weeks following the initial management of this patient's chylothorax there is persistent accumulation of chyle in the pleural space. Appropriate management at this time includes which of the following procedures?

(A) Neck exploration and ligation of the thoracic duct
(B) Subdiaphragmatic ligation of the thoracic duct
(C) Thoracotomy and repair of the thoracic duct
(D) Thoracotomy and ligation of the thoracic duct
(E) Thoracotomy and abrasion of the pleural space

Questions 396–397

A 43-year-old man suffers extensive injuries in a motor vehicle accident. Early in his course he has a tracheostomy. Six weeks later he has an episode of acute hemorrhage of approximately 150 ml of bright red blood from his tracheostomy.

396. Correct initial management of the patient described above would involve

(A) removal of the tracheostomy tube and oral endotracheal intubation
(B) continuous suctioning of the tracheostomy tube and emergency operative exploration
(C) packing of the pretracheal space with gauze
(D) repositioning of the tracheostomy tube and reinflation of the cuff
(E) none of the above

397. At the operation a trachea–innominate artery fistula is found and repaired. The innominate artery is ligated at its origin from the aorta and a 1-inch segment is removed. Following the procedure, the right arm will receive its blood supply from

(A) the suprascapular artery
(B) the internal thoracic artery
(C) the transverse cervical artery
(D) the axillary artery
(E) none of the above

DIRECTIONS: Each question below contains four suggested responses of which **one or more** is correct. Select

A	if	**1, 2, and 3**	are correct
B	if	**1 and 3**	are correct
C	if	**2 and 4**	are correct
D	if	**4**	is correct
E	if	**1, 2, 3, and 4**	are correct

398. Current contraindications to heart transplantation include

(1) colon cancer
(2) fixed pulmonary vascular resistance of 6 Woods units
(3) diverticulitis
(4) 55 years of age

399. The patient whose x-ray appears below is likely to develop

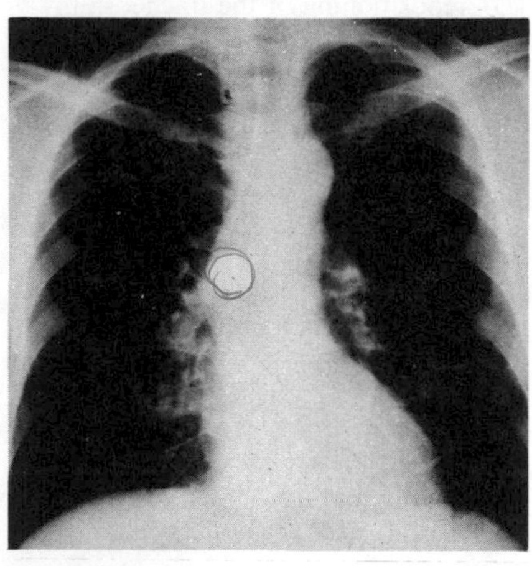

(1) atelectasis
(2) bronchiectasis
(3) a pulmonary abscess
(4) pneumothorax

400. Correct statements concerning aortocoronary bypass grafting include which of the following?

(1) It is indicated for crescendo (preinfarction) angina
(2) It is indicated for congestive heart failure
(3) It is indicated for chronic disabling angina
(4) It is associated with a 10 percent operative mortality

401. Correct statements concerning the thoracic outlet syndrome include which of the following?

(1) It may be difficult to distinguish from cervical spine disk disease
(2) It is reliably diagnosed by positional obliteration of the radial pulse
(3) If conservative measures fail, it is best treated by surgical decompression of the brachial plexus
(4) It most commonly affects the median nerve

402. Superior pulmonary sulcus carcinomas (Pancoast's tumors) are bronchogenic carcinomas that typically produce which of the following clinical features?

(1) Horner's syndrome
(2) Atelectasis of the involved apical segment
(3) Pain in the T1 and C8 dermatomes
(4) Nonproductive cough

---

403. The condition shown in the x-rays below is compatible with which of the following manifestations?

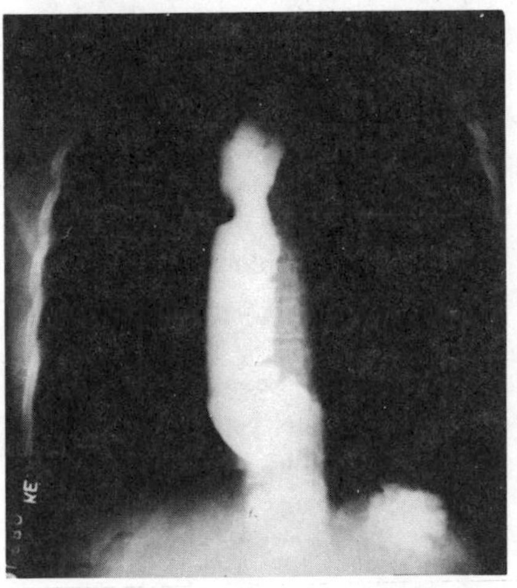

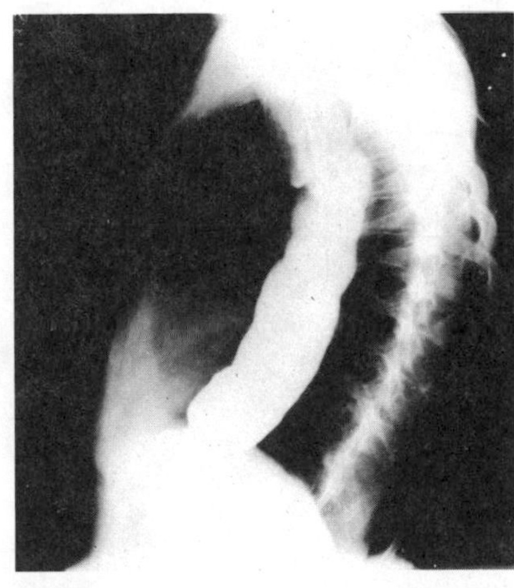

(1) Difficulty swallowing both solids and liquids
(2) Higher than normal incidence of esophageal carcinoma
(3) Failure of the lower esophageal sphincter to relax in response to swallowing
(4) Higher than normal pressure in the body of the esophagus

SUMMARY OF DIRECTIONS

A	B	C	D	E
1,2,3 only	1,3 only	2,4 only	4 only	All are correct

404. A 2-year-old asymptomatic child is noted to have a systolic murmur, hypertension, and diminished femoral pulses. Correct statements about this child's disorder include which of the following?

(1) The life expectancy without surgery is about 30 years
(2) Immediate surgery is indicated
(3) Rib notching is often seen on x-ray
(4) Claudication is frequently noted

405. A 35-year-old man presents with a history of 4 days of severe substernal pain and fever to 38.89°C (102°F). He has a past medical history of peptic ulcer disease that resulted in a Billroth II procedure 5 years earlier. On admission, the chest film below is obtained. True statements regarding this patient's case include which of the following?

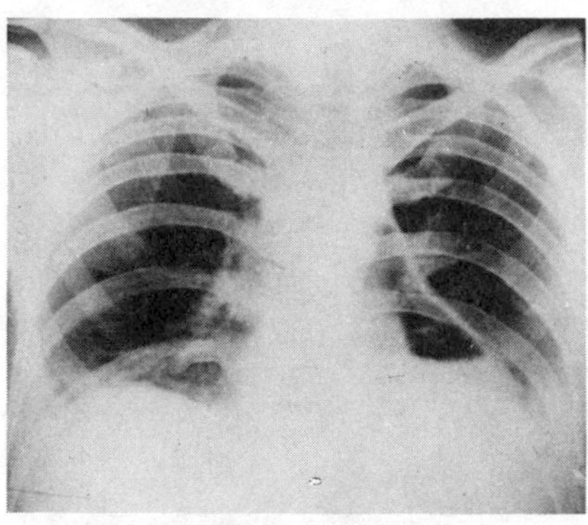

(1) Pneumopericardium is present
(2) The condition is a surgical emergency
(3) The condition could have resulted from recurrent peptic ulcer disease
(4) The condition could have resulted from spontaneous formation of gas from anaerobic bacteria

406. Correct statements concerning bronchial carcinoid tumors include that

(1) they infrequently metastasize
(2) they most commonly arise in the major proximal bronchi
(3) they rarely produce the carcinoid syndrome
(4) they are radiosensitive

407. Immunosuppressive agents used in the postoperative period following lung transplantation include

(1) azathioprine
(2) cyclosporine
(3) antilymphocyte globulin
(4) steroids

408. Generally accepted contraindications to surgery in the presence of a lung malignancy include which of the following?

(1) Extension of the tumor into the chest wall
(2) Paralysis of the phrenic nerve
(3) Pleural metastases
(4) Superior vena cava syndrome

DIRECTIONS: Each group of questions below consists of lettered headings followed by a set of numbered items. For each numbered item select the **one** lettered heading with which it is **most** closely associated. Each lettered heading may be used **once, more than once, or not at all.**

Questions 409–413

For each physical finding or group of physical findings below, select the cardiovascular disorder with which it is most likely to be associated.

(A) Massive tricuspid regurgitation
(B) Aortic regurgitation
(C) Coarctation of the aorta
(D) Thoracic aortic aneurysm
(E) Myocarditis

409. Conjunctivitis, urethral discharge, and arthralgia

410. Short stature, webbed neck, low-set ears, and epicanthal folds

411. Argyll Robertson pupil

412. Exophthalmos

413. Quincke's pulse

Questions 414–418

For each pathologic sign below, select the mediastinal tumor with which it is most likely to be associated.

(A) Thymoma
(B) Hodgkin's disease
(C) Neuroblastoma
(D) Parathyroid adenoma
(E) Cystic teratoma

414. T-cell deficiency

415. Ectopic hair

416. Increased urinary catecholamine level

417. Red blood cell aplasia

418. Renal stones

Cardiothoracic Problems
Answers

375. The answer is A. *(Schwartz, ed 5. p 432.)* Systemic evidence of cardiac transplant rejection is subtle, nonspecific, and frequently late. Endomyocardial biopsy is the preferred technique to identify early evidence of rejection and all patients undergo regular and fairly frequent endomyocardial biopsy of the right ventricle. Myocardial necrosis on biopsy is treated as rejection. Round cell infiltration should raise suspicion of rejection and warrants close follow-up. If diagnosis of rejection is delayed until arrhythmias or congestive failure develops, it is frequently irreversible.

376–377. The answers are: 376-B, 377-A. *(Sabiston, ed 4. pp 1067–1097.)* Ventricular septal defect accounts for 20 to 30 percent of all congenital cardiac anomalies. It may lead to cardiac failure and pulmonary hypertension if the defect is larger than 1 cm; or it may be completely asymptomatic if the defect is small. Surgery is not indicated for the asymptomatic patient with a small defect since a substantial number of these anomalies close spontaneously during the first few years of life. Operation is indicated in infants with congestive heart failure or rising pulmonary vascular resistance (owing to the left-to-right shunt). When symptoms are mild and can be controlled medically, operation is usually delayed until age 4 to 6. Operative mortality ranges from less than 5 percent to more than 20 percent depending on the degree of pulmonary vascular resistance. Tetralogy of Fallot, transposition, and tricuspid atresia are cyanotic lesions. Congenital cyanosis that persists beyond the age of 2 years is associated, in the vast majority of cases, with a tetralogy of Fallot. Patent ductus arteriosus is associated with the characteristic continuous machinery murmur.

378. The answer is B. *(Sabiston, ed 4. pp 1286–1291. Schwartz, ed 5. pp 870–875.)* Congestive heart failure in association with aortic stenosis signifies a reduction of left ventricular function and the end of compensatory cardiac reserve. Angina pectoris, syncope, exertional dyspnea, and palpitations, although ominous in their own right, tend to occur earlier in the course of aortic stenosis than does congestive heart failure. Even though cardiac compensation may be restored, once heart failure has occurred there is a high risk of sudden death, frequently during crisis periods. These crises, characterized by agitation, hyperhidrosis, flushing, and shock, are poorly understood.

379. The answer is C. *(Sabiston, ed 4. pp 418, 518, 521–522. Schwartz, ed 5. pp 743, 756.)* Hamartomas are common solitary lesions of pulmonary parenchyma that generally appear as asymptomatic coin lesions in the lung periphery. They consist of cartilage intermixed with other benign epithelial and mesodermal elements. Pulmonary chondromas arise from bronchial cartilage and are therefore more central; they often are endobronchial and produce signs and symptoms of bronchial obstruction. Teratomas (dermoid tumors) also contain cartilage but are cystic, usually contain hair, and usually occur in the mediastinum, gonads, and central nervous system. Since chondrosarcomas of the lungs are metastatic, it is probable that an affected patient would manifest symptoms of multiple lesions. Osteochondroma is a lesion of bone and is not found in pulmonary parenchyma.

380. The answer is B. *(Sabiston, ed 13. pp 767–773.)* Corrosive injuries of the esophagus most frequently occur in young children by accidental ingestion of strong alkaline cleaning agents. Significant esophageal injury occurs in 15 percent of patients with no oropharyngeal injury, while 70 percent of patients with oropharyngeal injury have no esophageal damage. Signs of airway injury or imminent obstruction warrant close observation and possibly tracheostomy. The risk of adding injury, particularly in a child, makes esophagoscopy contraindicated in the opinion of most surgeons. Administration of oral ''antidotes'' is ineffective unless given within moments of ingestion; even then, the additional damage potentially caused by the chemical reactions of neutralization often makes use of them unwise. A barium esophogram is usually done within 24 hours unless evidence of perforation is present. In most reports, steroids in conjunction with antibiotics reduce the incidence of formation of strictures from about 70 to about 15 percent. Vomiting should be avoided, if possible, to prevent further corrosive injury and possible aspiration. It is probably wise to avoid all oral intake until the full extent of injury is ascertained.

381. The answer is E. *(Sabiston, ed 4. pp 1586–1592. Schwartz, ed 5. pp 882–883.)* The patient described in the question manifests evidence of heart disease, a finding that is uncommonly associated with cardiac tumors other than myxomas. Myxomas are the most common primary cardiac tumors, constituting approximately half the primary tumors of the heart. Sarcomas account for about a quarter. Other primary tumors, such as hemangiomas and rhabdomyomas, are extremely rare. Malignant lymphoma and metastatic carcinoma, although usually asymptomatic and seldom seen except at autopsy, represent the most common of all cardiac neoplasms. Myxoma is a benign polypoid tumor that usually affects the left atrium. Because of its size, form, and location, the tumor compromises intracardiac blood flow and can mimic many primary cardiac diseases. While it does not invade contiguous structures nor does it metastasize, myxoma does tend to fragment and embolize. Hence, in atypical cases of acute arterial occlusion, such as in asymptomatic young patients who do not have a history of cardiac disease, histologic examination of emboli should be performed to rule out myxoma.

382. The answer is B. *(Sabiston, ed 4. pp 408–409. Schwartz, ed 5. pp 652–653.)* The most common cause of mediastinal emphysema in the adult is rupture of the esophagus. This may occur spontaneously (Boerhaave's syndrome), although most cases result from either diagnostic or therapeutic instrumentation. Pain caused by free air in the mediastinum can simulate the substernal pain associated with myocardial infarction, but careful auscultation of affected patients will usually reveal a loud crunching sound synchronous with the heartbeat (Hamman's sign). This is indicative of mediastinal emphysema. Because air within the mediastinum often is under tension, it may dissect into the pharyngeal tissues and mimic acute pharyngitis. While the pressure gradients leading to air dissection do not ordinarily allow tension to develop, if a traumatic ball valve (or flap valve) lesion in a major airway develops, sufficient pressure increase may interfere with venous return, and cyanosis and circulatory failure may ensue. Mediastinal emphysema may mimic heart failure in some ways, but the ventricles continue to deliver all the blood they receive—a low output state may develop, but it is not due to heart failure.

383. The answer is D. *(Sabiston, ed 4. pp 933–937.)* Although a systolic murmur is commonly heard with ventricular septal defect, atrial septal defect, congenital aortic stenosis, patent ductus arteriosus, and coarctation of the aorta, the hallmark of a patent ductus arteriosus is a continuous machinery murmur. It is a harsh rasping murmur that is loudest in systole and softest in diastole.

384. The answer is D. *(Schwartz, ed 5. pp 648, 686–687.)* In the x-ray shown in the question, tension pneumothorax is indicated by hyperlucency of the right hemithorax, a collapsed lung, and mediastinal shift to the opposite side. Because increased intrathoracic pressure and shift of the mediastinal structures can lead to cardiovascular collapse as a result of the decreased venous return, the situation may be life-threatening. Treatment, aimed at immediate reduction of the tension in the chest, is effected by insertion of either a 14-gauge needle into the pleural space or an intrapleural catheter attached to a water seal device. Elective thoracotomy is advisable for recurrent episodes of pneumothorax, for persisting air leakage, for large bullae or cystic lesions, and for refractory catamenial pneumothorax. The goal of treatment is pleurodesis (the production of adhesions between opposing pleural surfaces) to prevent the pleural space from filling with air. Positive-pressure ventilation before tube thoracostomy decompression could further increase the tension in the pleural space with catastrophic consequences. Bronchoscopy probably has no therapeutic role but may be useful for diagnostic purposes after control of the pneumothorax has been established.

385–386. The answers are: 385-D, 386-C. *(Sabiston, ed 4. pp 1286–1291. Schwartz, ed 5. pp 870–875.)* Aortic stenosis is associated with either rheumatic heart disease (in 30 to 50 percent of cases) or calcification of a congenitally bicuspid aortic valve. The onset of angina, syncope, or cardiac failure is ominous because death usually occurs within 2 years of the onset of failure and within 4 years following the onset of angina or syncope. Valve replacement is indicated in symptomatic patients and in those with an aortic valve gradient surpassing 50 mmHg. This procedure can be accomplished with a mortality of less than 10 percent.

387. The answer is C. *(Sabiston, ed 4. pp 1226–1245. Schwartz, ed 5. pp 855–866.)* Mitral stenosis almost always is a consequence of rheumatic fever. Stenosis of the valve leads to elevated left atrial pressures, atrial hypertrophy, atrial fibrillation, and thrombus formation along the atrial wall. Hemoptysis and tricuspid insufficiency are further consequences of the elevated pressure. Mitral commissurotomy or valve replacement is performed for symptomatic patients (dyspnea, orthopnea, hemoptysis, pulmonary edema, embolism, and angina).

388. The answer is E. *(Sabiston, ed 4. p 412. Schwartz, ed 5. p 763.)* Superior vena cava obstruction is almost always due to malignancy and, in three out of four cases, results from invasion of the vena cava by bronchogenic carcinoma. Lymphomas account for most of the remaining cases of the superior vena cava syndrome. Fibrosing mediastinitis as a complication of histoplasmosis or ingestion of methysergide may occur, but is rare. Rarely a substernal thyroid or thoracic aortic aneurysm may be responsible for the obstruction. Although constrictive pericarditis may decrease venous return to the heart, it does not produce obstruction of the superior vena cava. Whatever the cause of the superior vena cava syndrome, the resultant increased venous pressure produces edema of the upper body, cyanosis, dilated subcutaneous collateral vessels in the chest, and headache. Cervical lymphadenopathy may also be present, resulting from either stasis or metastatic involvement. When carcinoma is the cause of the superior vena cava syndrome, the treatment is usually palliative and consists of diuretics and radiation.

389. The answer is D. *(Sabiston, ed 4. pp 364–368. Schwartz, ed 5. pp 686–687.)* Spontaneous pneumothorax usually results from the rupture of subpleural blebs in young men (age 20 to 40), which is often signalled by a sudden onset of chest and shoulder pain. Pneumothorax of more than 25 percent requires placement of a chest tube; thoracotomy with bleb excision and pleural abrasion is generally recommended if spontaneous pneumothorax is recurrent. Small pneumothoraxes in patients with minimal symptoms usually resolve and therefore can be observed. A spontaneous perforation of the esophagus (Boerhaave's syndrome) can result in hydropneumothorax as well as the more usual pneumomediastinum, but would not present with an isolated 40 percent pneumothorax. Barium swallow is an appropriate diagnostic test for evaluation of a suspected leaking esophagus.

390. The answer is D. *(Schwartz, ed 5. p 648.)* Patients who have suffered blunt trauma sufficient to produce flail segments of the chest often develop severe hypoxemia. Though some references suggest that the paradoxical movement of the flail segment produces mechanical problems with ventilation that impair pulmonary ventilation, it is more likely that the underlying pulmonary contusion is the major cause of hypoxemia in these patients. When hypoxemia occurs, the preferred treatment is endotracheal intubation and positive pressure ventilation. The application of positive pressure ventilation to a seriously injured chest should probably be accompanied by the insertion of chest tubes into both pleural spaces, particularly in a hypotensive, unstable patient. The hypotension in this patient is presumably the consequence of hypovolemia. Most anesthetic agents cause a peripheral vasodilation, which could be fatal in this case. Ketamine, with sympathomimetic properties, is a notable exception. Muscle blockers can also cause hypotension by histamine release. The worst offender is curare; the safest is probably pancuronium. All victims of deceleration injuries should be presumed to have unstable cervical fractures until proved otherwise. For this reason some trauma surgeons prefer nasotracheal intubation. It is probably safe, however, to intubate the patient orally if axial traction is applied to the head during intubation.

391. The answer is B. *(Sabiston, ed 4. pp 399–402. Schwartz, ed 5. pp 683–686.)* There is no known association between mesotheliomas and previous thoracic trauma. A strong association exists, however, between mesothelioma and exposure to asbestos fiber. A similar high risk exists for the development of bronchogenic carcinoma. Both types of malignancy, which are associated with industrial or environmental exposure to asbestos, present a markedly increased risk in persons who also have a smoking history. Pain and swelling of joints, clubbing of the digits, and hypertrophic pulmonary osteoarthropathy all are manifestations of several intrathoracic disorders, including suppurative processes, lung tumors, and pleural tumors. A variety of extrapancreatic tumors, including mesotheliomas, occasionally cause hypoglycemia; the pathophysiology underlying this manifestation is unclear.

392. The answer is C. *(Sabiston, ed 4. pp 299–301.)* Rupture of the thoracic aorta associated with closed chest trauma most commonly occurs in the proximal descending aorta just distal to the left subclavian artery near the attachment of the ligamentum arteriosum. The mechanism of injury is believed to be rapid movement of the transverse arch against the relatively fixed descending aorta.

393. The answer is E. *(Schwartz, ed 5. pp 1132–1135.)* Pharyngoesophageal (Zenker's) diverticulum is an outpouching of mucosa between the lower pharyngeal constrictor and the cricopharyngeus muscle. It is thought to result from an incoordination of cricopharyngeal relaxation with swallowing. These diverticula occur in elderly patients and more commonly on the left. The typical patient will present with complaints of dysphagia, weight loss, and choking. Others present with the effects of repeated aspiration, pneumonia, or chronic cough. A mass is sometimes palpable and a gurgle may be heard. Treatment is excision and division of the cricopharyngeus muscle, which can be done under local anesthesia in a cooperative patient. Esophagoscopy is dangerous because the blind pouch is easily perforated. Even though the pouch may extend down into the mediastinum, the origin of the diverticulum is at the cricopharyngeus muscle near the level of the bifurcation of the carotid artery.

394–395. The answers are: 394-D, 395-B. *(Schwartz, ed 5. pp 681–683.)* Chylothorax may occur after intrathoracic surgery, or it may follow malignant invasion or compression of the thoracic duct. Intraoperative recognition of a thoracic duct injury is managed by double ligation of the duct. Direct repair is impractical owing to the extreme friability of the thoracic duct. Injuries not recognized until several days after intrathoracic surgery frequently heal following the institution of a low-fat diet and either repeated thoracentesis or tube thoracostomy drainage. A low-fat, medium-chain triglyceride diet often reduces the flow of chyle. Failure of this treatment modality requires direct surgical ligation of the thoracic duct. This is best approached from below the diaphragm, regardless of the site of intrathoracic injury.

396–397. The answers are: 396-D, 397-B. *(Anderson, ed 8. Figs. 1–16, 2–8, 7–12D, 7–27, 9–10, 9–12. Schwartz, ed 5. p 746.)* Massive hemorrhage from a trachea–innominate artery fistula is a highly lethal complication that usually is the result of anterior erosion of the tracheostomy tube into the innominate artery. This complication is most likely to occur if the tracheostomy is placed below the fourth tracheal ring. Immediate treatment consists of repositioning of the tracheostomy tube and reinflation of the cuff. Removal of the tube is not recommended because visualization of the field is impaired by massive hemorrhage. Occasionally, direct finger pressure on the innominate artery against the sternum will control the hemorrhage while arrangements are made for operation. Following ligation of the innominate artery, the right arm will receive its blood supply via retrograde flow through existing vessels. These vessels must arise distal to the point of ligation and must anastomose with at least one other major artery. Such vessels include the internal thoracic artery, which communicates with the deep epigastric artery, and the carotid and vertebral arteries, which anastomose with the circle of Willis. Although the transverse cervical artery and the subscapular artery arise distal to the point of ligation of the innominate artery ligation, they do not anastomose with vessels capable of providing significant retrograde arterial flow.

398. The answer is A (1, 2, 3). *(Schwartz, ed 5. pp 426, 427.)* Patients with active infections or neoplastic processes are not candidates for transplantation. Immunosuppression will exacerbate both processes. The pulmonary vascular resistance (PVR) must be evaluated carefully in the potential recipient of a heart transplant. A heart from a normal donor will fail if placed in a circuit with a fixed elevated vascular resistance. Any patient with a sustained pulmonary systolic pressure of 50 mmHg or greater is suspect. PVR is calculated by dividing the difference between the mean pulmonary artery pressure and wedge pressure by the cardiac index. This is expressed in Woods units and normal is between 0 and 3. If the PVR remains above 5 after infusion of nitroprusside or prostaglandin E-1, the risk of right heart failure in the transplant is excessive. Most transplant centers use age exclusion criteria. For most centers, 55 years of age is within the range in which transplantation would be done if a suitable donor could be found. However, this is a relative contraindication primarily based on consideration of allocation of scarce donor hearts.

399. The answer is A (1, 2, 3). *(Sabiston, ed 4. pp 68–70. Schwartz, ed 5. pp 704–708.)* The patient whose x-ray is presented in the question was a banker who, for reasons not entirely explained, made a deposit (a nickel) into his right bronchus. Though not a plug nickel, nickels do plug: this patient was in danger of developing atelectasis, pneumonitis, and lung abscess. If left on deposit, the investment would pay off by the development of bronchiectasis as a result of chronic partial bronchial obstruction. Pneumothorax is an unlikely complication of this patient's condition because the pleura is in no danger of penetration. The patient's chest film exhibits developing infiltrates in the distal parenchyma.

400. The answer is B (1, 3). *(Sabiston, ed 4. pp 1424–1445. Schwartz, ed 5. pp 887–891.)* Coronary artery bypass surgery was developed in the late 1960s and is now being regularly performed. Indications for surgery include chronic disabling angina and crescendo (or preinfarction) angina. Cardiac catheterization with selective coronary angiography defines the extent of disease, which generally is localized to the proximal segments of the vessels. Operative mortality is about 2 percent and relief of angina is obtained in most affected patients. Patients with left main coronary artery disease have an increased longevity following successful bypass. Data regarding extension of life in other groups of bypassed patients are conflicting.

401. The answer is B (1, 3). *(Sabiston, ed 4. pp 437–451.)* The thoracic outlet syndrome designates a symptom complex whose precise cause is unknown. It is felt to result from compression of the brachial plexus or subclavian vessels, or both, in the anatomic space bounded by the first rib, the clavicle, and scalene muscles. Since objective determinants of disease may be lacking or imprecise, the diagnosis often is established by resectional surgery. The carpal tunnel syndrome—compression of the median nerve as it passes through the carpal tunnel of the wrist—and cervical disk disease are the two entities most commonly confused with the thoracic outlet syndrome, whose symptoms and signs include pain, paresthesias, edema, venous congestion, and digital vasospastic changes. Positional dampening or obliteration of the radial pulse is an unreliable finding since it is present in up to 70 percent of the normal population. Neurologic abnormalities may be documented by nerve conduction studies. Angiographic studies are often negative. Conservative management, which generally should precede surgery, consists of an exercise program to strengthen shoulder girdle muscles and decrease shoulder droop. Operative treatment includes division of the scalenus anticus and medius muscles, first rib resection, cervical rib resection, or a combination of all three.

402. The answer is B (1, 3). *(Sabiston, ed 4. pp 506–514. Schwartz, ed 5. p 726.)* Pancoast's tumors are peripheral bronchogenic carcinomas that produce symptoms by involvement of extrapulmonary structures adjacent to the cupula. These structures include the nerve roots of C8 and T1, as well as the sympathetic trunk. Interruption of the cervical sympathetic trunk leads to miosis, ptosis, and anhydrosis, the triad of signs constituting Horner's syndrome. Involvement of the nerve roots causes pain along the corresponding dermatomes. The peripheral location of the neoplasm makes pulmonary signs, such as atelectasis and cough, unlikely.

403. The answer is E (all). *(Sabiston, ed 4. pp 720–721, 745–747.)* The x-rays presented in the question are consistent with a diagnosis of achalasia, a motility disorder of the esophagus that usually affects persons between 30 and 50 years of age. The x-rays show a classic beaklike narrowing of the distal esophagus and a large, dilated esophagus proximal to the narrowing. The diagnosis of achalasia is generally suspected on the basis of barium x-rays, but because other esophageal disorders may mimic the condition, an esophageal motility study is usually required to confirm the diagnosis. The characteristic findings on a motility study are small-amplitude, repetitive, simultaneous postdeglutition contractions in the body of the esophagus, failure of the lower esophageal sphincter to relax after deglutition, and a higher than normal pressure in the body of the esophagus. Carcinoma of the esophagus is approximately seven times more frequent in persons who have achalasia than in the general population.

404. The answer is B (1, 3). *(Sabiston, ed 4. pp 940–946.)* Coarctation of the aorta is a congenital anomaly that usually causes aortic stenosis just distal to the left subclavian artery in the area of the ligamentum arteriosum. Collateral circulation develops around the obstruction by way of intercostal vessels and accounts for the classic x-ray appearance of rib notching. Without surgery, the average life span is about 30 to 40 years with death resulting from cardiac failure, rupture of aortic aneurysms or of a cerebral artery, and bacterial endocarditis. Surgery can be accomplished with less than a 1 percent mortality and should be performed around 5 years of age, when the aorta is sufficiently large to be operable but before it becomes fibrotic and calcified, conditions that increase the technical difficulty of the operation.

405. The answer is E (all). *(Cummings, Ann Thorac Surg 37:511–518, 1984. Meyer, J Thorac Surg 17:62–71, 1948.)* This x-ray demonstrates an air-fluid level in the pericardium. Pneumopericardium can result from penetrating or blunt chest trauma, spontaneous formation of gas from anaerobic bacteria, iatrogenic causes, or direct extension into the pericardium by diseased adjacent organs. In this case, a patient with a high gastrojejunostomy developed a recurrent ulcer that eroded through the diaphragm and into the pericardium, thus causing a pneumopyopericardium. Often these patients will have an unrecognized gastrinoma (Zollinger-Ellison syndrome) and therefore continue to have peptic ulcer disease despite aggressive surgical therapy. The presence of pneumopyopericardium as seen in this chest film should be treated as a surgical emergency in this setting. Inability to demonstrate a fistula on roentgenographic investigation should not preclude the diagnosis of this entity. If the cause of the pericardial fluid is not clearly diagnosed by available means, then a pericardial window should be performed for diagnostic as well as therapeutic reasons. The pericardial sac should be irrigated and adequate continuing drainage should be ensured.

406. The answer is A (1, 2, 3). *(Schwartz, ed 5. p 723.)* Bronchial carcinoid tumors rarely produce the carcinoid syndrome. They are slow growing, infrequently metastatic tumors that histologically resemble the carcinoid tumors of the small intestine. Over 80 percent arise in the major proximal bronchi and their intraluminal growth is responsible for the frequent presentation of bronchial obstruction. The only therapy for this lesion is operative resection since neither the primary tumor nor the infrequent lymph node metastasis is radiosensitive. The low malignant potential for this lesion is reflected by a long-term survival rate that approaches 90 percent.

407. The answer is A (1, 2, 3). *(Schwartz, ed 5. pp 439–440.)* Early attempts at single lung transplantation were invariably fatal, ordinarily from early failure of the bronchial anastomosis. The Toronto group found that failure of this anastomosis was related to administration of steroids. They attribute their recent success to avoidance of steroids in the first 3 weeks after transplantation. They also construct a pedicle flap of omentum that surrounds and assists in the revascularization of the bronchial anastomosis. Their protocol includes cyclosporine, azathioprine, and ALG in the early postoperative period. Their favorable results have rekindled enthusiasm for clinical lung transplantation and a substantial increase in the clinical application of this technique can be anticipated in the next few years.

408. The answer is C (2, 4). *(Schwartz, ed 5. p 736.)* Paralysis of the phrenic nerve, vocal cord paralysis, and the superior vena cava syndrome are generally accepted contraindications to surgery for a primary lung malignancy because they usually indicate extensive tumor involvement of vital vascular structures. Pleural metastases and extension of the tumor into the chest wall are not absolute contraindications to surgery.

409–413. The answers are: 409-E, 410-C, 411-D, 412-A, 413-B. *(Sabiston, ed 4. pp 941, 971–972, 1211–1222.)* Myocarditis, aortitis, and pericarditis all have been described in association with Reiter's syndrome; the original description included conjunctivitis, urethritis, and arthralgias. Although its cause is unknown, Reiter's syndrome is associated with HLA-B27 antigen, as are aortic regurgitation, pericarditis, and ankylosing spondylitis.

Short stature, webbed neck, low-set ears, and epicanthal folds are the classic features of patients who have Turner's syndrome. Persons affected by the syndrome, which is commonly linked with aortic coarctation, are genotypically XO. However, females and males have been described with normal sex chromosome constitutions (XX, XY) but with the phenotypic abnormalities of Turner's syndrome. Additional cardiac lesions associated with Turner's syndrome include septal defects, valvular stenosis, and anomalies of the great vessels.

The Argyll Robertson pupil, a pupil that constricts with accommodation but not in response to light, is characteristic of central nervous system syphilis and is associated with vascular system manifestations of this disease. *Treponema pallidum* invades the vasa vasorum, causing an obliterative endarteritis and necrosis. The resulting aortitis gradually weakens the aortic wall, predisposing it to aneurysm formation. Once an aneurysm has formed, the prognosis is grave.

Massive *isolated* tricuspid regurgitation produces a markedly elevated venous pressure, usually manifested by a severely engorged (often pulsating) liver. If the venous pressure is sufficiently elevated, exophthalmos may result. Tricuspid regurgitation of rheumatic origin is almost never an isolated lesion, and the major symptoms of patients who have rheumatic heart disease usually are attributable to concurrent *left* heart lesions. Bacterial endocarditis from intravenous drug abuse is becoming an increasingly important cause of isolated tricuspid regurgitation.

Quincke's pulse, consisting of alternate flushing and paling of the skin or nail beds, is associated with aortic regurgitation. Other characteristic features of the peripheral pulse in aortic regurgitation include the water-hammer pulse (Corrigan's pulse—caused by a rapid systolic upstroke) and pulsus bisferiens, which describes a double systolic hump in the pulse contour. The finding of a wide pulse pressure provides an additional diagnostic clue to aortic regurgitation.

414–418. The answers are: 414-B, 415-E, 416-C, 417-A, 418-D. *(Sabiston, ed 4. pp 413–424. Schwartz, ed 5. pp 753–755.)* Thymomas are associated with myasthenia gravis, agammaglobulinemia, and red blood cell aplasia. These tumors are typically cystic and occur in the anterior mediastinum. Most thymic lesions associated with myasthenia gravis are hyperplastic rather than neoplastic.

Patients afflicted with Hodgkin's disease have impaired cell-mediated immunity and are particularly susceptible to mycotic infections and tuberculosis. The severity of the immune deficiency correlates with the extent of the disease. The nodular sclerosing variant of primary mediastinal Hodgkin's disease is the most common type.

Neuroblastoma, a highly malignant tumor of children, occurs along the distribution of the sympathetic nervous system. It is derived from ganglion cell precursors and thus usually causes an increased excretion of catecholamines and their metabolites. Because of its propensity to metastasize to bone and its histologic resemblance to Ewing's sarcoma, its association with elevated catecholamine levels is a major factor in differential diagnosis.

Renal stones occur in about half the cases of hyperparathyroidism. Other disorders sometimes associated with hyperparathyroidism include peptic ulcers, pancreatitis, and bone disease; central nervous system symptoms also may arise in connection with hyperparathyroidism. Occasionally, parathyroid adenomas occur in conjunction with neoplasms of other endocrine organs, a condition known as multiple endocrine adenomatosis.

Cystic teratomas, or dermoid cysts, include endodermal, ectodermal, and mesodermal elements. They characteristically are cystic and contain poorly pigmented hair, sebaceous material, and occasionally teeth. Dermoid cysts occur in the gonads and central nervous system, as well as in the mediastinum. With rare exceptions, the lesion is benign.

Peripheral Vascular Problems

DIRECTIONS: Each question below contains five suggested responses. Select the **one best** response to each question.

419. Patients with phlebographically confirmed deep vein thrombosis of the calf

(A) can expect asymptomatic recovery if treated promptly with anti-coagulants
(B) may be effectively treated with low-dose heparin
(C) may be effectively treated with pneumatic compression stockings
(D) may be effectively treated with acetylsalicyclic acid
(E) are at risk for significant pulmonary embolism

420. In renovascular hypertension, the most reliable indication of surgical correctability is

(A) the angiographic demonstration of significant arterial stenosis
(B) the demonstration of renin being produced solely by the involved kidney
(C) a positive split-renal function (Stamey or Howard) test
(D) an initial delay in the appearance and concentration of contrast medium in the involved kidney during intravenous urography
(E) a diastolic bruit in the flank over the involved kidney

421. A previously healthy 16-year-old high school student begins to notice pain in his right calf during football practice after running two laps around the track. The pain is relieved immediately when he stops running. The most likely diagnosis is

(A) arterial embolus
(B) muscle cramps
(C) popliteal entrapment syndrome
(D) popliteal aneurysm
(E) deep venous thrombosis

422. Venous ulceration of the lower extremity is caused chiefly by

(A) decreased greater saphenous vein flow
(B) arteriovenous shunting
(C) chronic venous hypertension
(D) hemosiderin deposition
(E) superficial varices

423. A 25-year-old woman presents to the emergency room complaining of redness and pain in the right foot up to the level of the midcalf. She reports that her right leg has been swollen for at least 15 years, but her left leg has been normal. On physical examination she has a temperature of 39°C (102.2°F). Her left leg is normal. The right leg is not tender, but it is swollen from the inguinal ligament down and she has an obvious cellulitis of her foot. Her underlying problem is

(A) popliteal entrapment syndrome
(B) acute arterial insufficiency
(C) primary lymphedema
(D) deep venous thrombosis
(E) none of the above

424. A 55-year-old man with recent onset of atrial fibrillation presents with a cold pulseless left lower extremity. He complains of left leg paresthesia and is unable to dorsiflex his toes. Following a successful popliteal embolectomy, with restoration of palpable pedal pulses, he is still unable to dorsiflex his toes. The next step in his management should be

(A) electromyography (EMG)
(B) measurement of anterior compartment pressure
(C) elevation of the left leg
(D) immediate fasciotomy
(E) application of a posterior splint

425. The angiogram depicted below is most typical of the patient whose history includes

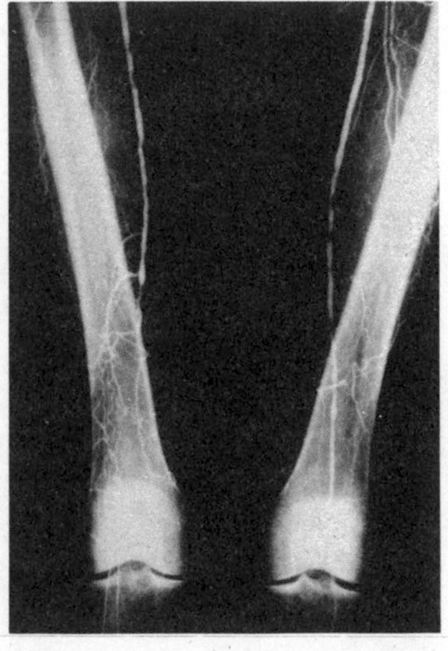
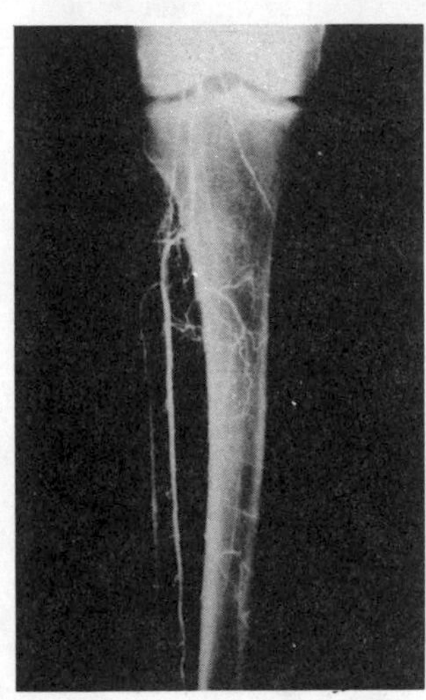

(A) cigarette smoking
(B) alcoholism
(C) hypertension
(D) diabetes
(E) type I hyperlipoproteinemia

---

426. Reconstructive arterial surgery rather than conservative management is generally recommended for patients with all the following symptoms or signs of arterial insufficiency EXCEPT

(A) ischemic ulceration
(B) ischemic neuropathy
(C) claudication
(D) nocturnal foot pain
(E) toe gangrene

427. Signs of chronic arterial insufficiency of the lower extremity include all the following EXCEPT

(A) loss of hair on the toes
(B) dependent rubor
(C) thickening of the toe nails
(D) brawny induration of the skin
(E) temperature difference between the foot and the thigh

428. A 48-year-old cirrhotic, alcoholic man is admitted via the emergency room with upper gastrointestinal hemorrhage. Bleeding is controlled with a Blakemore-Sengstaken tube after endoscopy confirms bleeding from esophageal varices. The transfusion requirement was 7 units. Physical examination reveals massive ascites and a midline abdominal scar that resulted from the need for a splenectomy (following trauma) some 3 years previously. In order to prevent further variceal bleeding the most appropriate surgical intervention would be an elective

(A) distal splenorenal shunt (Warren)
(B) mesocaval (H-graft) shunt
(C) end-to-side portacaval shunt
(D) side-to-side portacaval shunt
(E) end-to-end portacaval shunt

429. A 70-year-old man is found to have an asymptomatic abdominal mass and an arteriogram is obtained, which is pictured below. This patient should be advised that

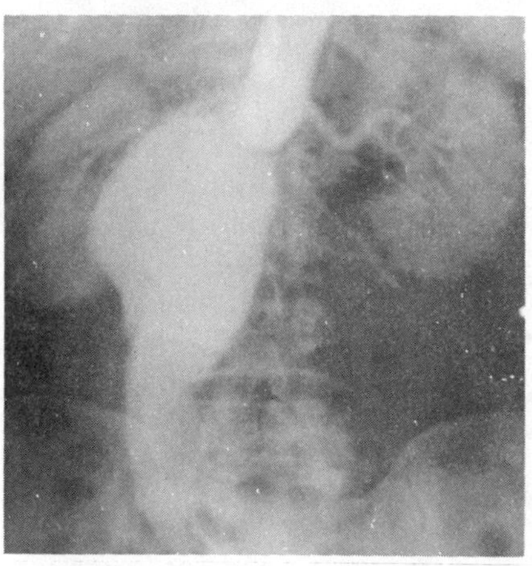

(A) surgery should be performed, but a mortality of 20 percent is to be anticipated
(B) surgery should be performed only if symptoms develop
(C) surgery will improve his 5-year survival
(D) surgery this extensive should not be performed in a patient of his age
(E) surgery should be performed only if follow-up ultrasound demonstrates increasing size

DIRECTIONS: Each question below contains four suggested responses of which **one or more** is correct. Select

A	if	**1, 2, and 3**	are correct
B	if	**1 and 3**	are correct
C	if	**2 and 4**	are correct
D	if	**4**	is correct
E	if	**1, 2, 3, and 4**	are correct

430. A 55-year-old man is scheduled to undergo elective coronary artery bypass, and during evaluation an asymptomatic right carotid bruit is discovered. An aortic arch angiogram is obtained, which is pictured below. This patient should be informed that

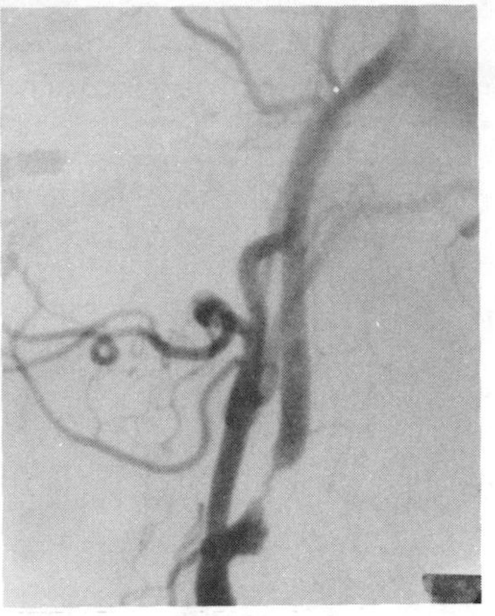

(1) he has a stenosis of the right internal carotid artery
(2) he should undergo carotid endarterectomy just prior to coronary artery bypass surgery in order to prevent an intraoperative stroke
(3) he may eventually develop transient ischemic attacks because of emboli from this stenotic, irregular internal carotid artery
(4) about 50 percent of patients suffer a stroke as the first symptom of carotid artery disease

431. Correct statements concerning antiplatelet therapy include

(1) aspirin has been shown to be an effective antiplatelet agent
(2) most antiplatelet agents work by inhibiting prostaglandin synthesis
(3) antiplatelet agents are used clinically in an attempt to increase patency rates of coronary artery bypass grafts
(4) it can be used to treat deep venous thrombophlebitis

432. Atherosclerotic occlusive disease of the lower extremities is more likely

(1) to be segmental than diffuse
(2) to be proximal than distal
(3) than coronary artery disease to progress rapidly
(4) than coronary artery disease to present with concomitant occlusive disease in other arterial beds

433. A 60-year-old man is admitted to the coronary care unit with a large anterior wall myocardial infarction. On his second hospital day he begins to complain of the sudden onset of numbness in his right foot and an inability to move his right foot. On physical examination the right femoral, popliteal, and pedal pulses are no longer palpable. Vascular consultation is obtained. Diagnosis of acute arterial embolus is made. Correct statements concerning this condition include

(1) appropriate management would be embolectomy of the right femoral artery under general anesthesia
(2) noninvasive hemodynamic testing is required
(3) prophylactic exploration of the contralateral femoral artery should be done despite the presence of a normal pulse
(4) the source of the embolus is most likely the left ventricle

434. The subclavian steal syndrome is associated with which of the following hemodynamic abnormalities?

(1) Reversal of flow through a vertebral artery
(2) Occlusion of a vertebral artery
(3) Occlusion of the subclavian artery
(4) Upper extremity venous congestion

435. True statements regarding pulmonary thromboembolism include which of the following?

(1) It is associated with clinically apparent deep vein thrombosis in less than 33 percent of patients
(2) It is believed to originate in deep vein thrombosis of the lower extremities in 85 to 90 percent of cases
(3) It causes hypoxemia owing to a ventilation-perfusion imbalance
(4) It must occlude more than 20 percent of the pulmonary vascular bed to produce symptoms in a previously healthy patient

436. Endarterectomy of the internal carotid artery is usually indicated in the presence of

(1) high-grade internal artery stenosis and history of transient ischemic attacks
(2) the stroke-in-evolution
(3) selected stable strokes
(4) severe intracranial arterial disease

437. Among patients with suspected (occult) coronary artery disease, the occurrence of postoperative ischemic cardiac events following peripheral vascular surgery correlates closely with abnormal preoperative

(1) exercise stress testing
(2) gated blood pool studies
(3) coronary angiography
(4) dipyridamole-thallium imaging

SUMMARY OF DIRECTIONS

A	B	C	D	E
1,2,3 only	1,3 only	2,4 only	4 only	All are correct

438. A 50-year-old male construction worker in relatively good health complains of severe left hip and left lower extremity pain that limits his walking radius to 100 feet. The angiogram pictured below was obtained. Therapeutic options in this patient include

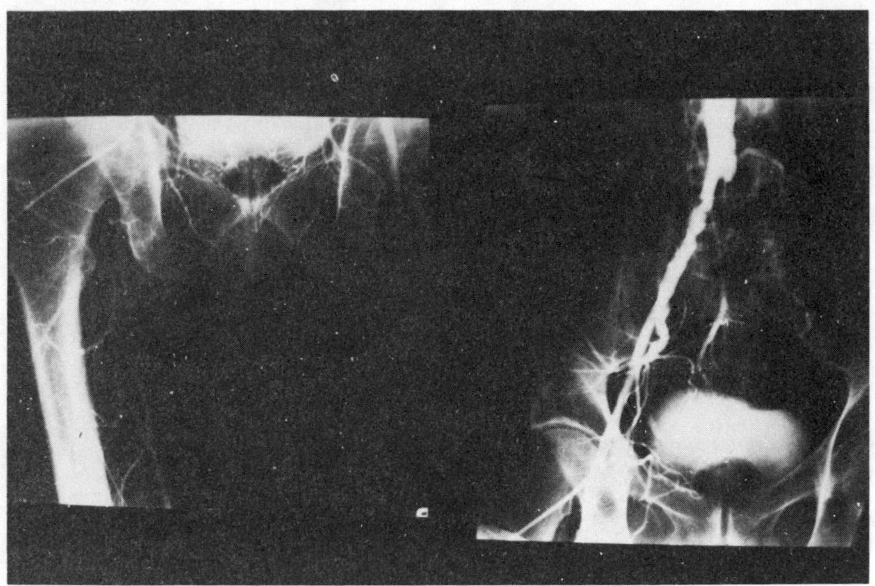

(1) femorofemoral bypass
(2) aortobifemoral bypass
(3) aorto–left-femoral bypass
(4) femoropopliteal bypass

439. A 65-year-old male cigarette smoker reports onset of claudication of his right lower extremity approximately 3 weeks previously. His walking radius is limited to three blocks before the onset of claudication. Physical examination reveals palpable pulses in his entire left lower extremity, but no pulses are palpable below the right groin level. Noninvasive flow studies are obtained, which are pictured below. Correct statements regarding this patient's condition include which of the following?

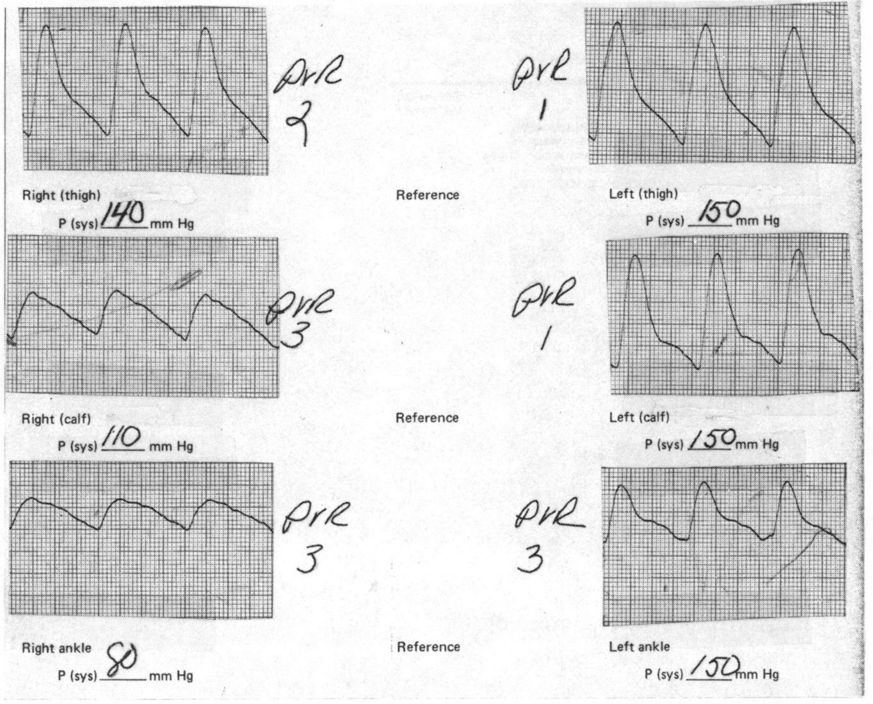

(1) Operative therapy (i.e., femoropopliteal bypass) is indicated on a relatively urgent basis in order to salvage the right leg
(2) The occlusive process is in the right superficial femoral artery with flow to the right foot being supplied by the profunda femoris artery
(3) The majority of patients with similar symptoms will ultimately require amputation
(4) The occlusive process is most likely on the basis of atherosclerotic disease

440. True statements concerning the condition depicted on the arteriogram shown below include which of the following?

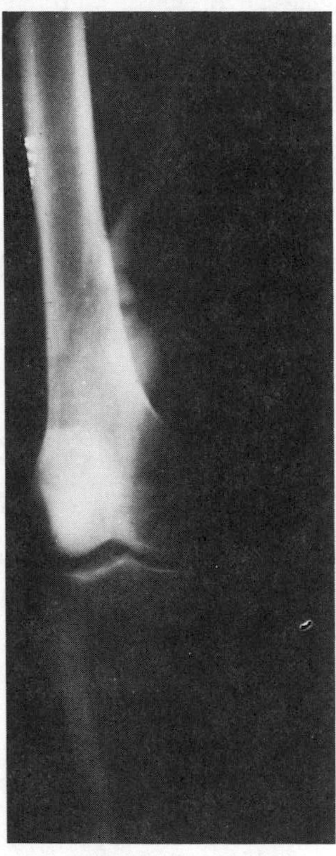

(1) Surgery should be performed even if the patient is asymptomatic
(2) Limb loss is a definite risk in the untreated patient
(3) The contralateral limb is often similarly affected
(4) Embolization is unlikely

441. Indications for placement of the device pictured in the abdominal x-ray shown below include

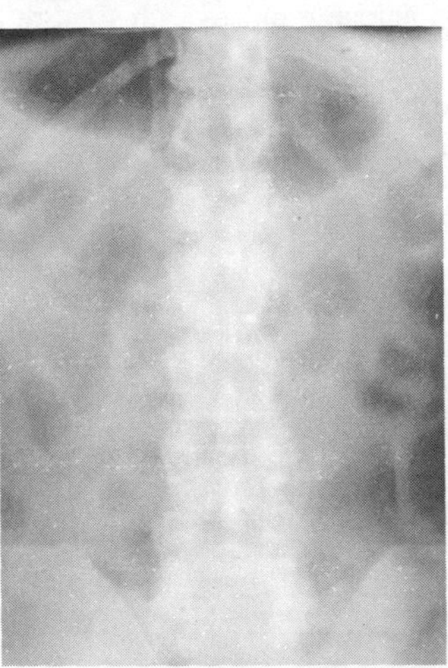

(1) recurrent pulmonary embolus despite adequate anticoagulation therapy
(2) axillary vein thrombosis
(3) pulmonary embolus occurring in a patient with a bleeding duodenal ulcer
(4) pulmonary embolus due to deep vein thrombosis of the lower extremity occurring 2 weeks postoperatively

442. Correct statements regarding Raynaud's disease include which of the following?

(1) The cause is unknown
(2) It more commonly affects women
(3) Vasoconstriction is usually precipitated by exposure to cold
(4) The upper extremities are almost always symmetrically involved

Peripheral Vascular Problems

Answers

419. The answer is E. *(Bergqvist, pp 69–77, 89–111, 120–123. Lindner, J Vasc Surg 4:436–442, 1986.)* Low-dose heparin and pneumatic compression stockings have been shown to be effective prophylaxis against deep vein thrombosis; however, they are not effective against established thrombosis, the treatment for which is therapeutic heparinization. Salicylate has not been convincingly shown to have either a prophylactic or therapeutic role in the treatment of deep vein thrombosis. Even following prompt, aggressive treatment of deep vein thrombosis of the calf as many as half of affected patients will develop symptoms of chronic venous hypertension, and a larger number will have abnormal venous hemodynamic findings. Untreated vein thrombosis of the calf may propagate into the larger popliteal veins and cause life-threatening pulmonary embolism.

420. The answer is B. *(Schwartz, ed 5. pp 1045–1058.)* Although atherosclerosis of the main renal arteries is often found at autopsy even in normotensive patients, surgically correctable atherosclerotic lesions account for less than 5 percent of cases of systemic hypertension in adults. Selection of patients for surgery requires a sensitive screening test (hypertensive excretory urography) as well as the demonstration of a correctable lesion (renal arteriography). However, the hypertension is curable only if it is maintained by unilateral renin production by the involved kidney. If the contralateral kidney has developed significant small-vessel arteriosclerosis and is also releasing renin, correction of the main renal arterial lesion will not cure the hypertension. The source of renin is determined by renal vein catheterization and measurement of bilateral renal venous (RV) and lower inferior vena caval (IVC) plasma renin activities. Surgical curability is predicted by unilateral excess renin production (involved/uninvolved RV renin ratio greater than 1.5) coupled with suppression of renin release by the uninvolved kidney (uninvolved RV/lower IVC ratio not greater than 1). While a unilateral flank bruit and a positive split-renal function test suggest the presence of a physiologically significant lesion, they do not reliably predict the response to surgery.

421. The answer is C. *(Rutherford, ed 2. pp 670–674.)* Claudication in young adults should suggest a popliteal entrapment syndrome because this congenital anomaly is the most common cause of claudication in this age group. The symptoms result from a compression of the popliteal artery, which passes medial to the medial head of the gastrocnemius muscle. The incidence of bilaterality is 25 percent. Operative repair is indicated once the diagnosis is made and includes dividing the medial head of the gastrocnemius muscle and repair of the artery if necessary. Arterial emboli do not generally present as claudication. Popliteal aneurysms may present as claudication but are rarely seen in this age group unless associated with an underlying entrapment.

422. The answer is C. *(Schwartz, ed 5. pp 1029–1035.)* Ulcers secondary to chronic venous insufficiency are the result of sustained hypertension in the superficial venous system. They are more commonly found in patients with deep venous abnormalities and incompetent perforating veins than in patients with primary varicose veins. These ulcers are usually located in the lower leg above the medial malleolus and over the incompetent perforating veins. At this location, extreme venous hypertension may occur as a result of the pumping effect of the muscles as they contract within the tight fascial compartments of the lower leg. Localized fibrosis and decreased vascularity, which develop as a result of the chronic high venous pressure, retard healing and predispose to both spontaneous skin breakdown and progressive ulceration following minor trauma. Treatment must be directed to correcting the underlying venous hypertension and to local wound care. Conservative management includes leg elevation and compression stockings. If the deep venous system is patent, excision of the varicose superficial veins with ligation of incompetent perforators may be indicated.

423. The answer is C. *(Rutherford, ed 2. pp 1450–1460.)* This patient is at high risk for developing cellulitis of her right foot because her underlying problem is unilateral primary lymphedema. Hypoplasia of the lymphatic system of the lower extremity accounts for greater than 90 percent of patients with primary lymphedema. If edema is present at birth it is referred to as congenital, but if it starts early in life (as in this woman) it is called praecox, and if it appears after age 35 it is tarda. The inadequacy of the lymphatic system accounts for the repeated episodes of cellulitis that these patients experience. Swelling is not seen with acute arterial insufficiency or with popliteal entrapment syndrome. Deep venous thrombophlebitis will result in tenderness and is generally not a predisposing factor for cellulitis of the foot.

424. The answer is D. *(Haimovici, ed 2. pp 1063–1070.)* This case illustrates two (among many) conditions leading to the anterior compartment syndrome, namely, acute arterial occlusion without collateral inflow, and rapid reperfusion of ischemic muscle. Treatment for a compartment syndrome is prompt fasciotomy. Assessing a compartment syndrome and proceeding with fasciotomy are generally based on clinical judgment. Inability to dorsiflex the toes is a grave sign of anterior compartment ischemia. EMG studies and compartment pressure measurements would probably be abnormal, but are unnecessary in view of the known findings and would delay treatment. Mere elevation of the leg would be an ineffective means of relieving compartment pressure, although elevation should accompany fasciotomy. Application of a splint has no role in the acute management of this problem.

425. The answer is A. *(Schwartz, ed 5. pp 965–967.)* The angiogram presented in the question demonstrates an isolated segment of atherosclerotic occlusion of the superficial femoral artery. Patients who have isolated femoropopliteal disease tend to be smokers, whereas those who have isolated tibioperoneal disease frequently are diabetic. Hypertension and hyperlipidemia predispose to accelerated atherosclerosis. On the other hand, type I hyperlipoproteinemia (hyperchylomicronemia), which is associated with dramatic levels of plasma triglyceride and formation of xanthomas, does not cause accelerated vascular disease.

426. The answer is C. *(Schwartz, ed 5. pp 957–972.)* The major threat to patients with arterial occlusive disease is limb loss. Ischemic ulceration, neuropathy, rest pain, and gangrene represent advanced stages of arterial insufficiency and warrant reconstructive surgery whenever clinically feasible. Claudication, in most cases, reflects mild ischemia; the majority of affected patients are successfully managed without surgery (only 2.5 percent develop gangrene). Most will stabilize or improve with development of increased collateral blood flow following institution of a program of daily exercise, cessation of smoking, and weight loss. Vasodilator drugs have been shown to have little benefit in the conservative management of intermittent claudication.

427. The answer is D. *(Rutherford, ed 2. pp 4–7.)* The signs of chronic arterial insufficiency result from chronic ischemia of the lower extremity. They include loss of hair on the dorsum of the toes, thickening of the toe nails, temperature difference between the foot and the thigh, painless ulcers on the distal aspect of the foot, and dependent rubor. Primary induration is a sign of chronic venous insufficiency in patients with a past history of deep venous thrombophlebitis.

428. The answer is D. *(Davis, pp 1606–1609.)* This patient cannot undergo a distal splenorenal shunt because a spleen is necessary for decompression of the varices via the short gastric vessels. The side-to-side portacaval shunt is the most attractive alternative because it will be more effective in reducing his ascites than the end-to-side portacaval shunt and has a higher patency than the interposition graft (mesocaval shunt).

429. The answer is C. *(Schwartz, ed 5. pp 981–988.)* Most abdominal aortic aneurysms are asymptomatic and are discovered on palpation by a physician. A radiograph of the abdomen is useful in demonstrating the aneurysm if there is calcification in the walls. Ultrasound is generally the first diagnostic procedure in confirming the presence of an aneurysm with arteriography performed if the aneurysm is considered large enough to require resection (greater than 5 cm in diameter). Recently CT scan has been useful as a preoperative study in patients suspected of having aneurysms. Surgery should be performed despite the absence of symptoms and can be carried out with a mortality of less than 5 percent. With leaking or ruptured aneurysms, the operative mortality associated with this emergency situation is upwards of 75 percent. The patient's age is not a contraindication to surgery since several studies have demonstrated a low mortality (less than 5 percent) and satisfactory long-term survival and quality of life in elderly, even octogenarian, patients.

430. The answer is B (1, 3). *(Barnes, Stroke 12:497–500, 1981. Davis, pp 2096–2103. Rutherford, ed 2. p 426.)* The treatment of the asymptomatic carotid bruit remains controversial. Agreement is fairly complete that patients with transient ischemic attacks (TIA) caused by extracranial vascular disease (i.e., internal carotid artery stenosis and/or plaque ulceration) should undergo carotid endarterectomy to reduce the probability of stroke. Most patients with carotid disease experience a TIA as the first symptom rather than a stroke. A study by Barnes and Marszalek has suggested that the presence of an asymptomatic carotid bruit does not increase the risk of intraoperative stroke during cardiac surgery, and therefore there is not urgent need to perform carotid endarterectomy in this asymptomatic patient prior to coronary bypass surgery.

431. The answer is A (1, 2, 3). *(Rutherford, ed 2. pp 302–303, 307–308.)* Aspirin exerts an antiplatelet effect that will last for the life of the platelet. Patients taking aspirin will experience its effect for 7 to 10 days after stopping the medication. Aspirin interferes with platelet function by inhibiting the synthesis of thromboxane A_2 and the subsequent production of prostaglandins. The platelet does not have a nucleus and thus cannot remanufacture the prostaglandins necessary for its functioning. Antiplatelet agents are generally used to prevent thrombotic and embolic events on the arterial side of the circulation. The Canadian Cooperative Study has shown antiplatelet therapy to be effective in preventing strokes in men with carotid artery disease, but it is not used to treat thrombophlebitis in the deep venous system. Antiplatelet therapy has been shown to increase graft patency rates following coronary artery bypass grafting if the medication is started preoperatively and continued postoperatively.

432. The answer is E (all). *(DeBakey, Ann Surg 201:115–131, 1985.)* Atherosclerotic occlusive disease tends to assume characteristic patterns that may be classified by predominant site or distribution of the disease: (I) the coronary artery bed; (II) branches of the aortic arch; (III) visceral branches of the abdominal aorta; (IV) the terminal aorta and its branches; and (V) combinations of I–IV. Disease in all categories tends to be well localized (segmental) and usually occurs in the proximal or midproximal portions of the arterial bed. Occlusive disease in the distal portions of the arterial bed is usually not amenable to effective surgical treatment. While all patients with atherosclerotic occlusive disease are at risk of developing new or recurrent critical lesions, patients with predominant involvement of the lower extremities or of the vessels of the aortic arch tend to be older, have disease that progresses faster, and have a higher incidence of concomitant occlusive lesions in other areas than patients with predominantly coronary or visceral artery disease.

433. The answer is D (4). *(Rutherford, ed 2. pp 449–459.)* The heart is the most common source of arterial emboli and accounts for 90 percent of cases. Within the heart, the sources include diseased valves, endocarditis, the left atrium in patients with unstable atrial arrhythmias, and mural thrombus on the wall of the left ventricle in patients having a myocardial infarction. The diagnosis in this patient is clear, and therefore noninvasive testing is not indicated. Arteriography is also not necessary and may prove to be too stressful for a patient undergoing an acute myocardial infarction. Embolectomy of the femoral artery can be performed under local anesthesia with minimal risk to the patient. Emboli typically lodge in one femoral artery and contralateral exploration is not indicated in the absence of signs or symptoms.

434. The answer is B (1, 3). *(Haimovici, ed 2. pp 223–230.)* Atherosclerotic occlusion of the subclavian artery proximal to the vertebral artery is the anatomic situation that results in the subclavian steal syndrome. On being subjected to exercise the involved extremity (usually left) develops relative ischemia, which gives rise to reversal of flow through the vertebral artery with consequent diminished flow to the brain. The upper extremity symptom is intermittent claudication. Venous occlusive disease is not a feature of the syndrome. The operative procedure for treating the subclavian steal syndrome consists of delivering blood to the extremity by creating either a carotid-subclavian or axillo-axillary bypass.

435. The answer is E (all). *(Hardy, ed 2. pp 1002–1015. Schwartz, ed 5. pp 1021–1027.)* Although the vast majority of pulmonary emboli are believed to originate in deep vein thrombosis of the legs (the remainder originating in the pelvic veins, right heart, and deep veins of the upper extremities), emboli in more than two-thirds of patients have clinically occult origins. A variety of diagnostic studies, using impedance plethysmography, radioactive-labeled fibrinogen, contrast venography, radionuclide (blood pool) venography, ultrasonography, and computed tomography, have been employed to identify the source of pulmonary emboli. While arteriovenous shunting in the lungs appears to play a role in the hypoxemia of pulmonary embolism, an increase in the ventilation-perfusion ratio of the affected areas, followed by reflex and, possibly, serotonin-mediated bronchoconstriction, is the main physiologic derangement. An otherwise healthy patient who has less than 20 percent of the pulmonary vascular bed occluded would remain asymptomatic and therefore would not be discovered without screening studies.

436. The answer is B (1, 3). *(Haimovici, ed 2. pp 800–801.)* Most stroke patients have a history of transient ischemic attacks (TIAs), and it is generally agreed that

TIAs are an indication for repair of arteriographically demonstrated carotid stenosis or ulcerated plaques. Correction of carotid occlusive disease is contraindicated in the patient with a large acute stroke because of the risk of conversion of an ischemic stroke to a hemorrhagic stroke and the attendant very high mortality. Under most circumstances, surgery is not indicated for an asymptomatic, incidentally noted carotid bruit or for patients with severe intracranial atherosclerotic arterial occlusive disease. Patients with acute mild strokes should be considered candidates for surgery.

437. The answer is C (2, 4). *(Boucher, N Engl J Med 312:389–394, 1985. Pasternack, Circulation 72:13–17, 1985.)* The occurrence of perioperative ischemic cardiac events among patients undergoing peripheral vascular reconstruction has been found to correlate with gated blood pool ejection fractions of 35 percent or less, and with reversible perfusion defects (thallium redistribution) on dipyridamole-thallium imaging. Ischemic rest pain or early onset of claudication after minimal exercise limits the effectiveness of stress testing as a screening procedure for occult coronary artery disease in this group of patients. Screening coronary angiography, followed by angioplasty or bypass of asymptomatic lesions, had an adverse effect on patient survival in a large prospective study of peripheral vascular surgery patients.

438. The answer is A (1, 2, 3). *(Schwartz, ed 5. pp 957–965.)* This patient has a total occlusion of the left common iliac artery. His symptoms are severe and limit his lifestyle and ability to earn a living, and therefore surgery is indicated. Therapeutic options include bypass from the aorta to the left common femoral artery or bypass to both common femoral arteries in the expectation that progression of disease will eventually cause problems on the currently uninvolved side. Femorofemoral bypass is also a reasonable option with an excellent long-term patency rate and the added advantage of not disturbing sexual function in this relatively young man. Dissection around the aorta will frequently result in a disturbance of the ejaculatory mechanism, which produces retrograde ejaculation. Femoropopliteal bypass or profundaplasty without correction of the iliac occlusion would be of no benefit to this patient.

439. The answer is C (2, 4). *(Schwartz, ed 5. pp 965–967.)* This patient has occlusion of the right superficial femoral artery caused by atherosclerosis, and this is confirmed by both physical examination and the flow study findings, which indicate a sharp decrease in the blood pressure below the level of the common femoral artery. Less than 10 percent of patients with claudication progress to gangrene and the need for amputation. Operative therapy would not be suggested at this time as it is quite likely that with cessation of cigarette smoking and adherence to an exercise program he could markedly improve his walking radius as collateral vessels enlarge to deliver more blood to the affected tissues. Operative therapy (femoropopliteal bypass) would be indicated at this time in this patient only if symptoms of rest pain or ischemic ulceration were present. Since physical examination and flow studies indicate disease distal to the aortoiliac distribution, aortoiliac reconstruction is not likely to be indicated in this patient.

440. The answer is A (1, 2, 3). *(Schwartz, ed 5. pp 988–989.)* Popliteal aneurysms are usually due to atherosclerosis, are bilateral 25 percent of the time, and require excision even if asymptomatic. Because of the risk of embolization (60 to 70 percent) and thrombosis with resultant gangrene, as well as the lesser risk of rupture, all of which lead to substantial likelihood of limb loss, even relatively small, asymptomatic aneurysms should be excised when discovered.

441. The answer is B (1, 3). *(Schwartz, ed 5. pp 1017–1019.)* The Greenfield filter pictured on the x-ray is used to interrupt migration of emboli to the lungs from the veins below the level of the filter. It is indicated in patients who sustain a recurrent pulmonary embolus despite adequate anticoagulant therapy or in patients with pulmonary emboli who cannot receive anticoagulants because of a contraindication (e.g., bleeding ulcer, intracranial hemorrhage). The filter is not used in patients who sustain a single pulmonary embolus. The filter is placed in the inferior vena cava just below the renal veins and therefore would not be effective for emboli that arise cephalad to its position.

442. The answer is E (all). *(Schwartz, ed 5. pp 996–1000.)* Vasospasm in the upper extremities initiated by exposure to cold or stress was described by Raynaud in 1862. It is now known that the condition can exist as a primary disorder (Raynaud's disease) or may be secondary to another disease (Raynaud's phenomenon). Associated conditions seen with Raynaud's phenomenon are thromboangiitis obliterans (Buerger's disease), scleroderma, cervical rib, atherosclerosis, disseminated lupus erythematosus, or periarteritis nodosa. The condition affects women (sex ratio of 5:1) and appears before age 40 in over 90 percent of patients. In the majority of patients, the episodes of vasoconstriction are precipitated by exposure to cold, but intense emotion has been noted as an inciting factor in some patients. The condition affects the upper extremities symmetrically, though in the minority of patients the lower extremities may also be affected. The findings of physical examination are usually normal in the early stages of the condition with ulcerations and punctate scars from healed ulcerations noted later as the disease progresses. When the condition is first noted, a thorough search for an underlying condition should be undertaken and the patient should be labeled as having primary Raynaud's disease only if no associated condition is discovered within 2 to 3 years after onset of symptoms. Treatment consists of avoidance of cold exposure and tobacco and the selective use of vasodilating drugs or intraarterial reserpine. Cervical dorsal sympathectomy with removal of the first, second, and third thoracic ganglia (preserving the cervical portion of the stellate ganglion to avoid a Horner's syndrome) has given excellent early results, but relapses are common. For this reason, sympathectomy is the therapy of last resort when symptoms are very severe and all other approaches have proved ineffective.

SPECIALTIES

Urology

DIRECTIONS: Each question below contains five suggested responses. Select the **one best** response to each question.

443. All the following statements regarding neuroblastoma are true EXCEPT that

(A) these tumors arise from the sympathetic nervous system and are usually found in the adrenal glands or posterior mediastinum
(B) 85 percent of tumors are discovered before the age of 3 years
(C) survival is very rare if osseous metastases are present
(D) survival is about the same as that seen in Wilms' tumor
(E) abdominal neuroblastoma is usually discovered as an irregular hard mass

Questions 444–445

444. A 3-year-old boy is found to be lacking a right testicle in his scrotum. The recommended management would be to

(A) follow the patient for several years
(B) institute a metastatic workup
(C) biopsy the descended testicle
(D) administer gonadotropins as soon as possible
(E) perform an orchiopexy as soon as possible

445. The patient in the preceding question is not seen again until 12 years of age when he complains of a swelling in his right groin. The most likely cause of the mass is

(A) testicular seminoma
(B) testicular torsion with necrosis
(C) thrombosis of the undescended spermatic vein
(D) acute epididymitis with edema
(E) metastatic neuroblastoma

446. A patient who has a flaccid neurogenic bladder may benefit initially from all the following measures EXCEPT

(A) being trained to void at timed intervals
(B) self-catheterization
(C) administration of bethanechol chloride (Urecholine)
(D) limiting fluid intake to less than 300 ml/day
(E) transurethral resection of the bladder neck

447. All the following statements concerning carcinoma of the prostate are true EXCEPT that it is

(A) the second most frequent cause of male cancer deaths in the United States
(B) more common among American blacks than other American ethnic groups
(C) associated with elevated serum acid phosphatase in about 60 percent of patients
(D) commonly asymptomatic in its early stages
(E) subject to control by estrogen therapy

DIRECTIONS: Each question below contains four suggested responses of which **one or more** is correct. Select

A	if	**1, 2, and 3**	are correct
B	if	**1 and 3**	are correct
C	if	**2 and 4**	are correct
D	if	**4**	is correct
E	if	**1, 2, 3, and 4**	are correct

448. A pedestrian is hit by a speeding car. Radiological studies obtained in the emergency room, including a retrograde urethrogram, are consistent with a pelvic fracture with a rupture of the urethra superior to the urogenital diaphragm. Management should consist of

(1) immediate placement of a suprapubic cystostomy tube
(2) immediate placement of a Foley catheter through the urethra into the bladder to align and stent the injured portions
(3) reconstruction of the ruptured urethra after 3 to 6 months to allow for resorption of the pelvic hematoma
(4) immediate exploration of the pelvis for control of hemorrhage from pelvic fracture and drainage of the pelvic hematoma

449. Correct statements regarding Wilms' tumors include which of the following?

(1) They generally present as an asymptomatic abdominal mass
(2) Chemotherapy is effective in this disease
(3) Nephrectomy with lymph node dissection is the preferred surgical treatment
(4) The incidence is greatest in the 5-to-10-year-old group of patients

450. Genitourinary tuberculosis in a male patient is suggested by which of the following findings?

(1) Microscopic hematuria
(2) Pyuria without bacteriuria
(3) Unilateral renal calcification
(4) Painless swelling of the epididymis

451. Correct statements regarding carcinoma of the prostate include which of the following?

(1) Bladder outlet obstruction is usually the presenting symptom
(2) Most tumors are unresectable by the time they are symptomatic
(3) Radionuclide scanning is a sensitive screening test for bony metastases
(4) Estrogen therapy significantly relieves pain in patients with bone metastases

452. Markers for testicular tumors include

(1) alpha-fetoprotein (AFP)
(2) testosterone
(3) beta subunit human chorionic gonadotropin (β-HCG)
(4) luteinizing hormone (LH)

SUMMARY OF DIRECTIONS

A	B	C	D	E
1,2,3 only	1,3 only	2,4 only	4 only	All are correct

453. During the course of an operation on an unstable, critically ill patient, the left ureter is lacerated through 50 percent of its circumference. If the patient's condition is felt to be too serious to allow time for definitive repair, alternative methods of management include

(1) ligation of the injured ureter and ipsilateral nephrostomy
(2) ipsilateral nephrectomy
(3) placement of a catheter from the proximal ureter through an abdominal wall stab wound
(4) placement of a suction drain adjacent to the injury without further manipulation that might convert the partial laceration into a complete disruption

454. A firm prostatic mass is discovered on rectal examination. Features of the mass suggestive of a malignant process would include

(1) indurated areas or nodules
(2) a rough irregular capsule
(3) elevated smooth or irregular borders
(4) adhesion and fixation to adjacent tissue

455. Seminoma is accurately described by which of the following statements?

(1) It is a common tumor of the testis
(2) Metastases to liver and bone are frequently found
(3) It is a very radiosensitive tumor
(4) The 5-year survival rate approaches 50 percent

Urology Answers

443. The answer is D. *(Schwartz, ed 5. pp 1720–1721.)* Neuroblastomas arise from the sympathetic nervous system and are typically found in the adrenal glands or posterior mediastinum. Younger children have a better prognosis; 50 percent of tumors are found in patients under 1 year of age and 85 percent in children under 3 years of age. The survival rate is 75 percent when tumors are discovered during the first year of life, even if there is metastatic spread to the bone marrow, liver, or skin; survival, however, is rare if there is evidence of osseous metastases. Evidence suggests that maternal immune factors are responsible for the improved survival in this younger age group. The abdominal tumors present as an irregular hard mass; intravenous pyelogram distinguishes these tumors from Wilms' tumors as there is no calyceal distortion with neuroblastoma. Surgical excision is the treatment of choice with adjuvant chemotherapy and radiotherapy usually recommended. Overall survival is not as good as that seen with Wilms' tumor.

444–445. The answers are: 444-A, 445-A. *(Schwartz, ed 5. pp 1717–1718.)* Nondescent of the testis into the scrotum (cryptorchidism) occurs in about 1 of every 20 full-term infants and 1 out of every 5 premature infants. If the testicle has not reached the scrotum by 6 weeks (3 months in premature infants), it probably will not spontaneously descend. Surgical placement in the scrotum (orchiopexy) should be accomplished before the child starts school and before active differentiation of the spermatocytic series begins—that is, when he is about 5 years of age. After the age of 6, irreversible damage may have taken place and the undescended testis may be permanently sterile.

Compared with descended testes, abdominal testes are 50 times more likely to develop neoplasms and those arrested in the inguinal canal have an elevenfold increase in risk of neoplastic transformation. Orchiopexy probably does not alter this incidence if the testicle did not spontaneously descend, but the procedure allows for closer examination of the testis. In view of the excessive risk, close regular follow-up is essential.

Seminomas are the most common type of testicular tumors associated with cryptorchidism, but teratomas and embryonal carcinomas are also found. It has also been established that a tumor is more likely to occur even in the descended testis of a unilaterally cryptorchid patient than in patients who have normally descended testes. Epididymitis and testicular torsion both produce pain but are unlikely to occur in an undescended testis. Metastatic neuroblastomas are very unusual malignancies of the testis. Spermatic vein thrombosis and cryptorchidism are not known to be associated with one another.

446. The answer is D. *(Schwartz, ed 5. pp 1741–1742.)* Patients who have a lower motor neuron lesion (flaccid neurogenic bladder) can usually be managed by conservative measures that prevent the development of a large residual urine volume in the bladder. These measures include intermittent self-catheterization and scheduled voiding with increased abdominal pressure provided by Valsalva's maneuver or manual pressure on the abdomen. Detrussor contractions can sometimes be strengthened by parasympathomimetic agents. Bladder neck resection may reduce outlet obstruction, but ureteral diversion is indicated only in the presence of gross ureterocalyxectasis that resists the foregoing measures. Severely restricting fluid intake is impractical and may promote formation of calculi.

447. The answer is E. *(Schwartz, ed 5. pp 1759, 1763–1768.)* Carcinoma of the prostate is second only to lung cancer as a cause of cancer death among men in the United States. It is nearly twice as common in American blacks as in American whites. In its earliest and most curable stages, carcinoma of the prostate is usually asymptomatic. Early detection depends on careful rectal examination, which should probably be performed regularly on men over 40 years of age. Serum acid phosphatase is elevated in about 60 percent of prostatic cancer patients and in approximately 80 percent of those who have bone metastases.

448. The answer is B (1, 3). *(Shires, ed 3. pp 358–361.)* If a rupture of the urethra is suspected, a retrograde urethrogram should be obtained *before* any attempts are made to place a Foley catheter, as efforts to do so may result in the creation of multiple false passages or conversion of a partial laceration into complete rupture. Previously, treatment had included attempts to realign the urethra immediately through the placement of interlocking sounds and traction using either a catheter passed over the sounds or perineal traction sutures through the bladder neck. Preferred treatment currently avoids either dissection into the pelvic hematoma surrounding the disruption or manipulation of the urethra; instead, only a suprapubic tube is placed immediately with delayed reconstruction after 3 to 6 months, at which time the hematoma will have resolved and the prostate will have descended into the proximity of the urogenital diaphragm.

449. The answer is A (1, 2, 3). *(Schwartz, ed 5. pp 1719–1721.)* Wilms' tumor is usually diagnosed after finding an asymptomatic mass in the upper abdomen. The sexes are equally affected, and age of onset is usually in the first 2 years of life. Diagnosis is usually confirmed by intravenous pyelogram, which demonstrates distortion of the collecting system. Patients with large tumors may have extension of the tumor to the renal vein or inferior vena cava. Nephrectomy with lymph node dissection is the preferred treatment with residual disease being treated with radiotherapy, actinomycin D, and vincristine. Wilms' tumor is one of the most curable cancers of childhood, with a 5-year survival of 80 percent. With tumor confined to the kidney or regional lymph nodes, the cure rate with surgery, chemotherapy, and radiotherapy is 95 percent.

450. The answer is E (all). *(Schwartz, ed 5. pp 1747–1748.)* Genitourinary tuberculosis develops from reactivation of foci in the renal cortex or prostate that were hematogenously seeded during the primary (usually asymptomatic) pulmonary infection. Local spread from the renal and prostatic sites can lead to involvement of the calyx, ureter, bladder, vas deferens, epididymis, and (rarely) the testis. A low-grade inflammatory response results in pyuria or hematuria. Whenever pus cells are seen on a routine urine culture without bacteria on smear or culture plate, genitourinary tuberculosis should be considered. The end result of focal caseation necrosis in the kidney may be scarring and dystrophic calcification. Genital tract infection often causes an asymptomatic swelling in the epididymis; secondary infection or formation of a sinus tract to the scrotal skin may cause more dramatic signs and symptoms.

451. The answer is E (all). *(Schwartz, ed 5. pp 1759, 1763–1768.)* Carcinoma of the prostate is a disease of older men and often coexists with benign prostatic hypertrophy. Ninety percent of prostatic carcinomas are unresectable by the time they block the prostatic urethra. The tumor spreads to vertebrae and the bony pelvis through the vertebral venous plexus, producing typical osteoblastic metastases. Although most prostatic carcinomas are hormone-dependent (stimulated to grow by androgens and inhibited by estrogens), controlled studies suggest that estrogen therapy does not prolong survival. Significant relief from the bone pain can be achieved by estrogen therapy, however, and many urologists accordingly reserve it for use in the symptomatic patient.

452. The answer is B (1, 3). *(Catalona, Surg Clin North Am 62:1119–1127, 1982.)* In patients with testicular carcinoma, AFP levels are elevated in approximately two thirds of the patients with advanced nonseminomatous tumors but not elevated in patients with seminoma or choriocarcinoma. β-HCG levels are elevated in about two thirds of patients with advanced nonseminomatous tumors and in 15 percent of patients with advanced seminomas. Almost all patients with choriocarcinoma have elevated β-HCG levels. If both AFP and HCG are measured, almost 90 percent of patients with advanced nonseminomatous tumors will have an elevation of either marker. In patients with minimal evidence of disease, the markers are much less reliable. HCG or AFP levels may be elevated in only 50 percent of patients with grossly normal appearing but histologically involved nodes (stage IIA). Therefore, retroperitoneal metastases or unsuspected distant metastases may be present in patients with normal CT scans and normal AFP and HCG levels. Luteinizing hormone and testosterone levels play no diagnostic or prognostic role in testicular tumors.

453. The answer is B (1, 3). *(Shires, ed 3. pp 354–355.)* If time and the patient's condition permit, primary ureteral reconstruction should be carried out. In the middle third of the ureter, this will usually consist of ureteroureterostomy using absorbable sutures over a stent. If the injury involves the upper third, ureteropyeloplasty may be necessary. In the lower third, ureteral implantation into the bladder using a tunneling technique is preferred. If time does not permit definitive repair, suction drainage adjacent to the injured segment alone is inadequate; either ligation and nephrostomy, or placement of a ureteral catheter is an acceptable alternative that would allow reconstruction to be performed later. The creation of a watertight seal is difficult and nephrectomy may be required if the injury occurs during a procedure in which a vascular prosthesis is being implanted (e.g., resection of an aortic aneurysm, aortoiliac bypass procedures) and contamination of the foreign body by urine must be avoided.

454. The answer is E (all). *(Schwartz, ed 5. pp 1759, 1763–1768.)* Several pathologic entities can present clinically as a solitary prostate mass and mimic prostatic carcinoma. These include the benign processes of prostatic infarction, granulomatous prostatitis, prostatic atrophy, and calcific nodules in the prostate. All the clinical signs listed in the question suggest the possibility of prostatic malignancy; further diagnostic evaluation is indicated whenever any of these signs is found.

455. The answer is B (1, 3). *(Schwartz, ed 5. pp 1768–1770.)* Seminomas tend to grow slowly and metastasize late. They represent about 40 percent of malignant testicular tumors; embryonal cell carcinomas and teratocarcinomas each represents about 25 percent. Since most tumors have mixed elements, they are usually classified according to the most malignant cell type encountered, whatever the predominant cell type. When metastases occur, they are usually along the regional lymphatic drainage pathways to the iliac, aortic, and renal lymph nodes. Because of their slow growth and radiosensitivity, seminomas are associated with a 90 percent 5-year survival rate. Therapy generally consists of removing the affected testis and sampling the lymph nodes (usually external iliac) for evidence of metastasis. If metastases are present, radiation therapy is given locally to areas of known involvement. Radiation therapy is highly effective in seminoma, and metastatic disease may be palliated for extended periods.

Orthopedics

DIRECTIONS: Each question below contains five suggested responses. Select the **one best** response to each question.

456. The most severe epiphyseal growth disturbance is likely to result from which of the following types of fracture?

(A) Fracture dislocation of a joint adjacent to an epiphysis
(B) Fracture through the articular cartilage extending into the epiphysis
(C) Transverse fracture of the bone shaft on the metaphyseal side of the epiphysis
(D) Separation of the epiphysis at the diaphyseal side of the growth plate
(E) Crushing injury compressing the growth plate

457. In an uncomplicated dislocation of the glenohumeral joint, the humeral head usually dislocates primarily in which of the following directions?

(A) Anteriorly
(B) Superiorly
(C) Posteriorly
(D) Laterally
(E) Medially

458. Which of the following statements regarding osteitis deformans (Paget's disease) is true?

(A) It occurs more frequently in males
(B) Pain is usually improved with repetitive exercise
(C) It is usually limited to a single bone
(D) Serum calcium and phosphorus are usually normal
(E) Spontaneous fractures are rare

459. Meniscal tears usually result from which of the following circumstances?

(A) Hyperextension
(B) Flexion and rotation
(C) Simple hyperflexion
(D) Compression
(E) Femoral condylar fracture

460. A march fracture most frequently arises as a consequence of which of the following circumstances?

(A) Direct trauma to the foot
(B) A twisting injury to the ankle
(C) Jumping onto a hard surface from a height
(D) Persistent use of high-heeled shoes
(E) Muscle fatigue

461. All the following anatomic features are associated with congenital talipes equinovarus (clubfoot) EXCEPT

(A) plantar flexion of the ankle
(B) adduction of the forefoot
(C) medial rotation of the tibia
(D) inversion of the foot
(E) hypoplasia of the calcaneus

DIRECTIONS: Each question below contains four suggested responses of which **one or more** is correct. Select

A	if	**1, 2, and 3**	are correct
B	if	**1 and 3**	are correct
C	if	**2 and 4**	are correct
D	if	**4**	is correct
E	if	**1, 2, 3, and 4**	are correct

462. In contrast with closed reduction, open reduction of a fracture causes

(1) a longer healing time
(2) increased trauma to the fracture site
(3) a higher incidence of nonunion
(4) a greater risk of infection

463. True statements regarding compartment syndromes following orthopedic injuries include which of the following?

(1) The first sign is usually loss of pulse in the extremity
(2) Passive flexion of the distal extremity will aggravate the pain
(3) Surgical decompression (fasciectomy) is necessary only as a last resort
(4) They are most commonly associated with supracondylar fractures of the humerus and tibial shaft

464. Correct statements about bones that have been fractured, properly aligned, and have healed include which of the following?

(1) They often regain their normal elasticity
(2) They often regain their normal strength
(3) They usually exhibit some degree of shortening
(4) They often regain their normal structure

DIRECTIONS: Each group of questions below consists of lettered headings followed by a set of numbered items. For each numbered item select the **one** lettered heading with which it is **most** closely associated. Each lettered heading may be used **once, more than once, or not at all.**

Questions 465–469

For each description below, select the type of fracture/dislocation with which it is most likely to be associated.

(A) Navicular fracture
(B) Monteggia's deformity
(C) Greenstick fracture
(D) Spiral fracture
(E) Posterior shoulder dislocation

465. Seen after epileptiform convulsion

466. Avascular necrosis not uncommon

467. Dislocation of the radial head and fracture of the proximal third of the ulna

468. Commonly occurs in young people who fall on an outstretched hand

469. Tenderness in the anatomist's snuffbox

Questions 470–473

For each of the conditions listed below, choose the fracture with which it is most likely to be associated.

(A) Colles' fracture
(B) Humeral shaft fracture
(C) Supracondylar fracture of the humerus
(D) Calcaneal fracture
(E) Supracondylar fracture of the femur

470. Volkmann's ischemic contracture

471. Median nerve injury

472. Compression fracture of the spine

473. Radial nerve injury

Questions 474–477

For each description below, select the bone lesion with which it is most likely to be associated.

(A) Osteoid osteoma
(B) Osteochondroma
(C) Osteosarcoma
(D) Aneurysmal bone cyst
(E) Unicameral bone cyst

474. X-ray may show periosteal elevation overlying the lesion and a "sunburst" appearance of subperiosteal bone; the most common presenting symptom is pain

475. Arises from the cartilaginous elements of developing bone; frequently asymptomatic

476. X-ray may show a round or oval defect in bone without adjacent reactive bone formation; the most common presenting symptom is pathologic fracture

477. Proliferation of vascular tissue in bone destroys the overlying bone cortex

Orthopedics
Answers

456. The answer is E. *(Schwartz, ed 5. p 1943.)* Longitudinal growth of bone follows ossification of cartilage that forms at the epiphyseal plate. Fractures that involve separation of the growth plate (type I) (almost always occurring on the diaphyseal side) may be realigned; normal growth usually follows epiphyseal separation because the proliferative cells are still attached to their blood supply in the bone epiphysis. Fractures extending perpendicular to and through the epiphysis (types II, III, IV) may result in the formation of bony bridges across the epiphysis that can disrupt later growth. Though all the fractures listed in the question place the epiphyseal growth plate in some jeopardy, crushing injuries to the epiphysis (type V) have the worst prognosis; numerous bony bridges may form and prevent longitudinal growth.

457. The answer is A. *(Schwartz, ed 5. pp 1948–1950.)* The glenohumeral joint is bounded posteriorly by the teres minor and infraspinatus muscles and partially by the long head of the triceps. It is bounded laterally by the powerful deltoid muscle; superiorly, the acromion process precludes upward dislocation. However, anteriorly and inferiorly the pectoralis major and the long head of the biceps do not completely stabilize the glenohumeral joint; in this region the articular ligaments and joint capsule provide the major structural support. Thus, the joint is not strongly supported in its anteroinferior aspect, and consequently anterior (or anteroinferior) dislocations are the most common glenohumeral dislocations. The humeral head is driven anteriorly, tearing the shoulder capsule, detaching the labrum from the glenoid, and producing a compression fracture of the humeral head. Most glenohumeral dislocations result from a posteriorly directed force on an arm that is partially abducted. Posterior dislocation is much rarer and should raise the possibility of a seizure as the precipitating cause.

458. The answer is D. *(Schwartz, ed 5. pp 1933–1934.)* Osteitis deformans was originally described in 1876 by Sir James Paget and is now known as Paget's disease. It is characterized by increased bone resorption with deposition of new bone in an irregular fashion. The bone changes consist of thickening, softening, and deformity followed by ossification. The cause of Paget's disease is unknown. It appears in the fourth to sixth decade, with an equal distribution between the sexes. A frequent presentation is pain in the lower extremities, which is often worse at night and aggravated by exercise. Paget's disease usually begins in a single bone, most commonly the tibia, but will progress to a generalized form involving multiple bones in over three quarters of the patients. The radiologic appearance reflects the stage of the disease. Serum calcium and phosphorus are usually normal, but alkaline phosphatase is elevated. Spontaneous fractures are a frequent complication and may occur with minimal trauma. A more ominous complication is the development of sarcomas in affected bone. There is as yet no satisfactory cure for Paget's disease, and therapeutic interventions are palliative.

459. The answer is B. *(Schwartz, ed 5. pp 1966–1967.)* Most meniscal tears are produced by flexion and rapid rotation. A classic example (''football knee'') involves a player who is hit while running. The knee, supporting all the player's weight, usually is slightly flexed and the foot is anchored to the ground by cleats. Impact from an opposing player usually causes rotation almost entirely restricted to the knee. The injury involves rapid rotation of the flexed femoral condyles about the tibial plateau, most frequently tearing the medial or, less frequently, the lateral meniscus. A tear in the inner free border of the cartilage is also common whenever excessive rotation without flexion or extension occurs. Early surgical removal of the displaced menisci is usually recommended to prevent further damage to the cartilage or ligaments.

460. The answer is E. *(Schwartz, ed 5. p 1974.)* A march fracture usually occurs in the shaft of the second or third metatarsal. It results from the stress of weight bearing after prolonged walking and probably is related to loss of muscular and tendinous support of the foot. Pain is usually not noticed until a week or more passes, at the time callus formation can be demonstrated on x-ray. Only rarely is there a history of direct trauma to the foot. Long-term use of high-heeled shoes may precede development of Morton's neuralgia (traumatic neuroma). Twisting injuries cause sprains or, if severe enough, ankle fractures. Jumping onto a hard surface from a height most often causes calcaneal fractures, but may also cause vertebral compression fractures and pelvic fractures.

461. The answer is E. *(Schwartz, ed 5. pp 1917–1918.)* The anatomic features of congenital talipes equinovarus (clubfoot) are plantar flexion of the ankle, inversion of the foot, adduction of the forefoot, and medial rotation of the tibia. There are no structural abnormalities of the bones initially, except for their altered relative position. Treatment should begin as early as possible and proceed in a systematic fashion. By the application of serial corrective casts, the adduction of the foot must be corrected first, followed by the inversion of the hindfoot, then the plantar flexion. If the foot is dorsiflexed prior to correction of the hindfoot varus, a rocker-bottom foot may be created. Most cases of clubfoot can be corrected in this fashion within a few weeks. More difficult cases may require operative correction.

462. The answer is E (all). *(Schwartz, ed 5. p 1944.)* Open reduction of a fracture involves the restoration of normal bone alignment under direct observation at surgery. In effect, open reduction converts a simple fracture into a compound (or open) fracture and thereby increases the risk of infection. Operative manipulation also increases trauma at the fracture site and may consequently add to the probability of infection. Hematomas at the site of fracture may be important for early healing; open reduction, which usually involves removing the clots in the field, could contribute to a delay in bone healing and to nonunion. The major advantage of open reduction is the shorter period of immobilization it allows, an advantage that often outweighs all the disadvantages previously mentioned, as in the open reduction of femoral neck fractures in the elderly. This allows these patients to get out of bed much sooner than if they were treated with several weeks of traction.

463. The answer is D (4). *(Schwartz, ed 5. pp 1952–1953, 1969–1970.)* Compartment syndromes result from increasing pressures in the fascial compartments of the arm or leg. When the pressure in the muscles is greater than that of the capillaries, ischemia and necrosis of the muscles occur even though the arterial pressure is still high enough to produce pulses; pulselessness is an unreliable sign. Extreme pain (out of proportion to the injury), pain on passive extension of the fingers or toes, pallor of the extremity, motor paralysis, and paresthesias are all components of the syndrome. The patient will usually hold the injured part in a position of flexion to maximally relax the fascia and reduce the pain; passive extension will usually produce severe pain. The diagnosis can be confirmed by measuring intracompartmental pressures, but whenever physical findings or symptoms are suspicious, immediate surgical decompression by fasciectomy is indicated since delay is likely to lead to irreversible damage.

464. The answer is C (2, 4). *(Schwartz, ed 5. pp 1938–1941.)* If a simple fracture is properly aligned, then over a long period of remodeling (up to 3 years) the bone should recover its normal strength and gross and microscopic structure. Normal tissue elasticity never returns to the fractured segment, even after prolonged remodeling and after both gross and microscopic evidence of fractures have disappeared. Although some fractures may cause shortening, most do not. For instance, in children they may stimulate the epiphyseal growth plates and actually cause overgrowth.

465–469. The answers are: 465-E, 466-A, 467-B, 468-A, 469-A. *(Schwartz, ed 5. pp 1946–1964.)* Fractures of the navicular of the wrist should be suspected in anyone, particularly young people, who falls on an outstretched hand. Although x-rays are mandatory, it is important to realize that the fracture may not be seen on the initial x-ray and that a presumptive diagnosis can and should be made on clinical grounds alone. Typically, there will be tenderness to palpation over the navicular tuberosity and limitation of wrist flexion and extension. Immobilization of the wrist for about 16 weeks and sometimes up to 6 months is required. Nonunion or avascular necrosis is not uncommon and may require bone grafting to correct.

Dislocation of the radial head with a fracture of the proximal third of the ulna is known as Monteggia's deformity. Usually, the radial head is dislocated anteriorly.

The injury is usually caused by forced pronation. The injury can be treated by reduction and stabilization of the ulna followed by reduction of the radial head via supination and direct pressure.

Anterior shoulder dislocations occur more frequently than posterior dislocations. However, posterior dislocations are seen in special situations, such as during an epileptiform convulsion and during electroshock therapy. Closed reduction followed by immobilization is usually sufficient therapy.

A spiral fracture, frequently seen in the tibia in skiers, results from the application of torque to a long bone. Greenstick fractures are common in children. The bones of young children are able to bend to a greater degree than those of adults; the fracture may occur only at the site of maximal cortical stress but not at the opposite cortex, the site of maximal longitudinal compression.

470–473. The answers are: 470-C, 471-A, 472-D, 473-B. *(Schwartz, ed 5. pp 1950–1964.)* Colles' fracture typically occurs in patients over 50 years of age who fall on an outstretched hand. Also called a silver-fork fracture, it was described by Abraham Colles in 1814. The x-ray appearance is that of a dorsally angulated fracture of the distal radial metaphysis, with an associated fracture of the ulnar styloid. The median nerve is at risk with this injury, and so a careful assessment of median nerve function must be documented.

Supracondylar fracture of the humerus is most often seen in children. It is usually caused by a fall on an extended elbow. The brachial artery may be injured, with resulting ischemia to the flexor forearm muscles that eventually results in Volkmann's contracture.

The radial nerve is the most commonly injured nerve in the humeral shaft fracture. Spontaneous recovery occurs in over 95 percent of cases without open reduction.

Fractures of the calcaneus most commonly occur after falls. Associated injuries occur in approximately 25 percent of these patients. These injuries include compression fractures of the spine, pelvis fractures, or lower extremity fractures.

Supracondylar fractures of the femur are intraarticular fractures since they have a communication with the knee. Long-term sequelae may involve difficulties with knee motion.

474–477. The answers are: 474-C, 475-B, 476-E, 477-D. *(Schwartz, ed 5. pp 670, 2003–2010.)* Osteosarcomas arise from osteoblasts and usually cause death within 2 years of diagnosis. They generally arise in long bones—particularly the femur—and initially cause pain. Later, local swelling and tenderness may appear. Overlying bone is irregularly eroded; the tumor may break the cortex and expand into adjacent soft tissue. Osteosarcomas may rise in bones affected by Paget's disease.

Osteoid osteoma also arises from osteoblasts but is usually seen in males in their teens or twenties. Night pain, which responds only to aspirin, is the classic presenting symptom. Treatment is resection of the lesion, which is usually in the lower extremity or the spine.

Osteochondromas, which are benign projections of bone covered by a cartilaginous cap, usually develop at the end of a long bone, most frequently from the tibia or femur near the knee. Arising during the second decade of life, they cease growing upon closure of the epiphyses and are asymptomatic unless they are subjected to trauma or impinge on sensitive tissue. Osteochondromas occasionally undergo malignant transformation.

Unicameral bone cysts are single-chambered, benign lesions, most frequently occurring as solitary lesions in the proximal humerus or femur. They frequently are associated with pathologic fractures because of thinning of adjacent bone cortices. The cysts do not undergo malignant transformation. Treatment consists of scraping the cyst walls and packing with bone chips or removal of the entire segment of bone containing a cyst (subperiosteal resection).

Aneurysmal bone cysts, thought to arise from vascular tissue in bone, frequently cause local pain. Pathologic fractures are commonly associated with these cysts and may be accompanied by heavy bleeding. Preferred surgical treatment consists of curettage and packing with bone chips. Radiation may induce vascular sclerosis in surgically inaccessible cysts.

Neurosurgery

DIRECTIONS: Each question below contains five suggested responses. Select the **one best** response to each question.

478. All the following statements regarding the Glasgow coma scale are true EXCEPT

(A) it serves as a scale to assess severity of head trauma
(B) a high score correlates with a high mortality
(C) it measures eye opening
(D) it measures motor response
(E) it measures verbal response

479. A 19-year-old woman with tetralogy of Fallot has an acute onset of fever, vomiting, dulled sensibility, and seizures. The most likely diagnosis is

(A) subdural hematoma
(B) epidural abscess
(C) brain abscess
(D) subdural empyema
(E) berry aneurysm

480. Ten years after radical mastectomy for breast carcinoma, a 55-year-old woman returns to her doctor with visual complaints; she has otherwise been feeling well. Skull x-rays reveal an area of destruction of the sella turcica, with small calcifications throughout the lesion. The most likely diagnosis is which of the following neoplasms?

(A) Pituitary adenoma
(B) Craniopharyngioma
(C) Chordoma
(D) Granular cell tumor
(E) Metastatic breast carcinoma

481. A 25-year-old man is brought to the emergency room and gives a history of sudden onset of severe headache. There is no history of loss of consciousness. Physical examination does not disclose any evidence of focal neurological deficit. The most likely diagnosis is

(A) subdural hematoma
(B) epidural hematoma
(C) meningioma
(D) berry aneurysm
(E) carotid artery occlusion

482. All the following statements regarding skull fractures are true EXCEPT that

(A) depressed fractures are those in which the cranial vault is displaced inward
(B) compound fractures are those in which the bone and the overlying skin are broken
(C) any bone fragment displaced more than 1 cm inwardly should be elevated surgically
(D) drainage of cerebrospinal fluid via the ear or nose requires prompt surgical treatment
(E) most skull fractures do not require surgical treatment

483. An 18-year-old man is admitted to the emergency room following a motorcycle accident. He is alert and fully oriented but witnesses to the accident report an interval of unresponsiveness following the injury. Skull films disclose a fracture of the left temporal bone. Following x-ray the patient suddenly loses consciousness and dilatation of the left pupil is noted. This patient should be considered to have

(A) a ruptured berry aneurysm
(B) acute subdural hematoma
(C) epidural hematoma
(D) intraabdominal hemorrhage
(E) ruptured arteriovenous malformation

484. Spontaneous subarachnoid hemorrhage is most frequently caused by which of the following abnormalities?

(A) Arteriovenous malformation
(B) Intracranial aneurysm
(C) Thromboembolism
(D) Atherosclerotic vascular disease
(E) Hypertension

485. True statements about acromegaly include all the following EXCEPT

(A) cardiac disease is a common cause of death
(B) the tumor secretes growth hormone
(C) growth-hormone–secreting cells originate in the neurohypophysis
(D) bitemporal hemianopsia is a common finding
(E) prolactin levels are frequently elevated

DIRECTIONS: Each question below contains four suggested responses of which **one or more** is correct. Select

A	if	**1, 2, and 3**	are correct
B	if	**1 and 3**	are correct
C	if	**2 and 4**	are correct
D	if	**4**	is correct
E	if	**1, 2, 3, and 4**	are correct

486. Correct statements regarding the condition suggested by the CT scan shown below include which of the following?

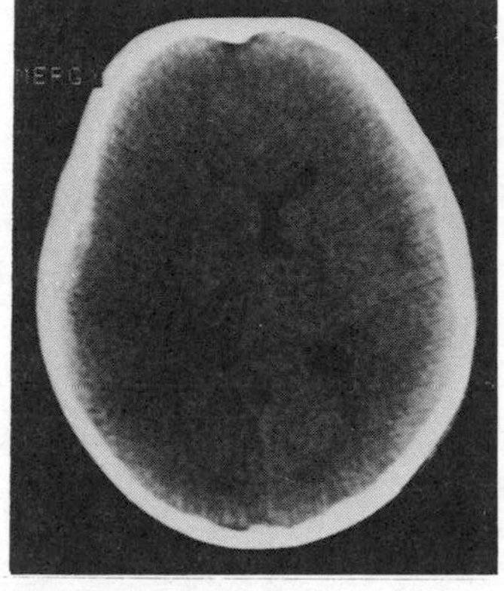

(1) It is caused by rupture of the veins traversing the subdural space
(2) Symptoms may occur at any time up to 2 months after injury
(3) Without treatment, the brainstem will be compressed by hemorrhage and edema with herniation, resulting in death
(4) The condition should be suspected in the presence of progressive change in mentation and a fluctuating level of consciousness

487. An epidural hematoma is likely to occur after which of the following head injuries?

(1) Contracoup injury to the occipital lobe
(2) Blunt temporal trauma
(3) A depressed frontal fracture
(4) A linear temporal-parietal fracture

488. Correct statements concerning craniopharyngiomas include which of the following?

(1) The tumors are frequently cystic
(2) The tumors are nearly always benign
(3) The tumors may cause compression of optic tracts and visual symptoms
(4) The tumors may cause ventricular obstruction and hydrocephalus

489. Correct statements regarding cerebral contusions include which of the following?

(1) They occur most frequently in the frontal lobes
(2) They may occur opposite the point of skull impact
(3) They are usually accompanied by bleeding
(4) They may cause subsequent neurologic disorders

SUMMARY OF DIRECTIONS

A	B	C	D	E
1,2,3 only	1,3 only	2,4 only	4 only	All are correct

490. A posterolateral herniation at the interspace between L4 and L5 may produce

(1) weakness of dorsiflexion of the great toe
(2) sensory deficit on the lateral aspect of the foot
(3) hyperesthesia on the dorsum of the foot
(4) weakness on plantar flexion

491. Increased intracranial pressure is characterized by which of the following clinical findings?

(1) Respiratory irregularities
(2) Increased blood pressure
(3) Bradycardia
(4) Decreased auditory acuity

492. Treatments that have proved beneficial for patients afflicted with neuroblastoma include

(1) resection
(2) chemotherapy
(3) irradiation
(4) immunosuppression

Neurosurgery Answers

478. The answer is B. *(Schwartz, ed 5. p 1838.)* The Glasgow coma scale was developed to assess the severity of head trauma. It measures the level of consciousness using three parameters: verbal response, motor response, and eye opening. The score is the sum of the highest number achieved in each category. The fully oriented and alert patient will receive a maximum score of 15. A score of less than 5 is associated with a mortality of over 50 percent.

479. The answer is C. *(Howard, ed 2. pp 469–474. Schwartz, ed 5. pp 1863–1865.)* The brain is resistant to infection by bacteria. It has been shown experimentally that, even with direct bacterial inoculation, it is difficult to create a brain abscess. The presence of underlying brain damage, such as hypoxia, trauma, or hemorrhage, facilitates the formation of an abscess. The dura mater itself is an effective barrier against infection. However, a weakness in the barrier exists at those points where somatic and cranial nerves penetrate the dura, thereby allowing an avenue to the central nervous system for bacteria. The causes of brain abscesses can be divided into three categories: (1) direct extension from an adjacent infection, e.g., from the middle ear, mastoid, and paranasal sinus; (2) hematogenous or metastatic spread; (3) direct traumatic penetration. Patients with a right-to-left cardiac shunt have a tenfold higher risk over the general population of developing a brain abscess because they lose the bacterial filtering capacity of the lung. Patients with tetralogy of Fallot are at even great risk because of the higher viscosity of the blood and reduced blood flow. The clinical picture of a brain abscess depends on its chronicity. The symptoms may vary from those of an acute systemic infection to those of a space-occupying mass lesion. Thus, a high index of suspicion is crucial for an early diagnosis of a brain abscess because the symptoms may be subtle and misleading. CT scan is the diagnostic test of choice. The goals of medical treatment are to control the infection with antibiotics and to reduce the cerebral edema with steroids. However, antibiotics may not be able to penetrate the abscess cavity and thus surgical drainage continues to be the definitive curative procedure.

480. The answer is B. *(Schwartz, ed 5. pp 1555–1557.)* Craniopharyngioma is a squamous cell tumor probably arising from embryonal remnants of Rathke's pouch. It usually is located in the suprasellar area but also may occupy the sella itself. Focal calcification is present in almost all cases; in about 75 percent of the cases, the calcification is prominent enough to appear on x-ray. Total excision is the primary treatment, but recurrence of the tumor is not uncommon. None of the other tumors listed in the question are characterized by this type of calcification, although pituitary adenomas often cause sella destruction. Granular cell tumors usually arise from the stalk or posterior lobe of the pituitary gland but rarely cause symptoms. Chordomas arise from remnants of the notochord, usually in the bone, and can affect areas from the sacrococcyx to the skull. In the skull, these tumors usually involve the spheno-occipital region and may encroach on the sella turcica. Metastases to the pituitary and sella from breast carcinoma, which are chiefly autopsy findings, may occasionally cause diabetes insipidus.

481. The answer is D. *(Schwartz, ed 5. pp 1859–1860.)* Subarachnoid hemorrhage occurring in the absence of a history of trauma suggests a ruptured berry aneurysm. Sudden headache or transient loss of consciousness occurs because of the intracranial hemorrhage. Other possible causes of these symptoms are hypertensive hemorrhage or bleeding from an arteriovenous malformation. The majority of intracranial aneurysms arise from the arteries of the circle of Willis and at the origin of large vessels from the vertebral-basilar system. Twenty percent of the aneurysms are multiple. Approximately 27 percent of patients die within the first week after rupture. A second hemorrhage (peak occurrence 7 to 12 days following the initial hemorrhage) carries a mortality of 42 percent. The likelihood of rebleeding diminishes significantly after 6 weeks. Therapy is directed at removing the aneurysm from the force of systolic blood pressure.

482. The answer is D. *(Schwartz, ed 5. pp 1836–1837.)* Most skull fractures do not require surgical treatment unless they are depressed or compound. A general rule is that all depressed skull fractures should be surgically elevated, especially if they are depressed more than 1 cm, if a fragment is over the motor strip, or if small sharp-appearing fragments are seen on x-ray (as they may tear the underlying dura). Compound fractures must be cleansed and debrided and the wound closed. When a skull fracture occurs in an area of the paranasal sinuses, mastoid air cells, or the middle ear, a tear in the meninges may result in cerebrospinal fluid drainage from the ear or nose. The presence of rhinorrhea or otorrhea requires observation and prophylactic antibiotics, as meningitis is a serious sequela. Otorrhea usually heals within a few days. Persistent cerebrospinal fluid from the nose or ear for more than 14 days requires surgical repair of the torn dura.

483. The answer is C. *(Schwartz, ed 5. pp 1841–1842.)* Epidural hematomas may be caused by either venous or arterial bleeding. The surgically important epidural hematomas are usually caused by arterial bleeding. Rupture of the middle meningeal artery caused by fracture of the temporal bone where the artery is adjacent to the bone is the most likely cause of the epidural hematoma. The typical history is one of head trauma followed by a momentary alteration in consciousness and then a lucid interval lasting for up to a few hours. This is followed by a loss of consciousness, dilatation of the pupil on the side of the epidural hematoma, and then compromise of the brainstem and death. Treatment consists of temporal craniectomy, evaluation of the hemorrhage, and control of the bleeding vessel. The mortality of epidural hematoma is approximately 50 percent.

484. The answer is B. *(Schwartz, ed 5. pp 1859–1860.)* Intracranial aneurysms account for more than half the cases of spontaneous subarachnoid hemorrhage. Other frequent causes are hypertension and atherosclerotic vascular disease (15 percent). It is possible that physical exertion, such as heavy lifting or sexual intercourse, may cause hemorrhage from aneurysms, although most cerebral aneurysms cause no clinical disease and are incidental findings at autopsy. Once rupture has occurred, the mortality is approximately 50 percent and recurrence of bleeding is common among survivors.

485. The answer is C. *(Schwartz, ed 5. pp 1548–1551, 1553.)* Growth-hormone–secreting cells are found in the lateral aspect of the adenohypophysis of the pituitary gland. Excess growth hormone in children produces gigantism and in the adult acromegaly. The main cause of excess production of growth hormone is a benign pituitary adenoma. As these tumors grow, they may compress the visual tracts at the optic chiasm and give rise to visual symptoms, most frequently bitemporal hemianopsia. The physical findings of enlarged face, hands, and feet are characteristic. Patients also have organomegaly, including cardiomegaly, which may result in valvular dysfunction and cardiomyopathy. Glucose and fat metabolism are altered in the presence of excess growth hormone. Diabetes mellitus and atherosclerosis are frequently present. Patients with pituitary tumors that secrete excess growth hormone frequently have elevated levels of prolactin, which results in galactorrhea and menstrual dysfunction in female patients.

486. The answer is E (all). *(Schwartz, ed 5. pp 1840–1841.)* Subdural hematoma is caused by rupture of the veins traversing the subdural space from the brain to the dural sinuses. The symptoms may occur within a few minutes or as long as 8 weeks after injury. With acute subdural hematoma, significant progressive neurologic deficit is noted within 48 hours of injury. Without treatment, the brainstem is compressed by hemorrhage and edema until herniation occurs, resulting in death. Computerized axial tomography is accurate in defining the site of recent intracranial hemorrhage. Treatment consists of craniotomy with removal of the hematoma and relaxation of the compressing dura. Mortality in this acute form of the condition is very high (up to 80 percent). Subacute subdural hematomas are defined as those that cause significant neurologic deficits more than 48 hours but less than 2 weeks after injury. Chronic subdural hematomas are those that cause symptoms 2 weeks or more after injury. They are most commonly seen in infants or elderly patients and are suggested by a change in mental faculties or a fluctuating or decreasing level of consciousness.

487. The answer is C (2, 4). *(Schwartz, ed 5. pp 1841–1842.)* Epidural hematomas usually are secondary to injury to the middle meningeal artery or to bleeding from dural sinuses or dural veins. While 90 percent of epidural hematomas are associated with linear skull fractures, these hematomas also occur in blunt head trauma without evidence of fracture. In patients who have had injuries requiring hospitalization, approximately 2 percent suffer epidural hematomas. Epidural hematomas are particularly apt to occur in association with an injury caused by sudden angular acceleration or a change in any diameter of the skull.

488. The answer is E (all). *(Schwartz, ed 5. pp 1555–1557.)* Craniopharyngiomas are usually benign pituitary tumors arising from the epithelium of Rathke's pouch. Frequently cystic, these neoplasms produce symptoms of compression, since they tend to expand rather than to invade. Compression of optic tracts may produce bitemporal hemianopsia and pressure upon the ventricular system may result in hydrocephalus. Treatment consists of simple excision (if the tumors are well encapsulated) or cyst drainage with partial resection.

489. The answer is E (all). *(Schwartz, ed 5. pp 1837–1842.)* The most frequent sites of cerebral contusions are the orbital surfaces of the frontal lobes and the frontotemporal junctions. Cerebral contusions may result from contracoup injury (injury opposite the point of skull impact—particularly occipital trauma). Bruising is always present, and subsequent neurologic impairment (epileptic disorders) is common if the original injury was significant (altered consciousness exceeding 4 hours in duration). Patients so affected should probably be protected by receiving anticonvulsive medications, at least during the early posttraumatic period.

490. The answer is B (1, 3). *(Schwartz, ed 5. pp 1887–1888.)* The intervertebral disc is subject to early degenerative changes, especially in the lower cervical and lower lumbar regions. These changes include thinning of the annulus fibrosus, loss of fibrocartilage, and dehydration of the nucleus pulposus. Herniation of portions of the disc can be a serious sequela of these degenerative changes. Not all herniations of the disc are symptomatic, but of those that are symptomatic, the highest incidence occurs in the lumbar region. These are usually unilateral, and 95 percent are found in the lower two interspaces. A posterolateral herniation in the lumbar region impinges on the anterior and posterior nerve roots of the caudad intervertebral foramen. Thus, a herniation at the interspace between L4 and L5 will compress the fifth lumbar roots. The anterior root of L5 serves the anterior crural and peroneal muscles, and the most common finding with its compression is weakness of dorsiflexion of the great toe. The posterior root of L5 serves the dermatome from the anterolateral aspect of the leg to the dorsum and medial aspect of the foot, and thus compression may present as hyperesthesia on the dorsum of the foot. Weakness on plantar flexion and sensory deficit on the lateral aspect of the foot are symptoms associated with compression of the first sacral roots, a sequela of posterolateral herniation at L5-S1.

491. The answer is A (1, 2, 3). *(Schwartz, ed 5. pp 1837–1852.)* Increased intracranial pressure causes systemic hypertension, bradycardia, and respiratory irregularities. Cheyne-Stokes respiration occurs more commonly than hyperventilation, although hyperventilation may result from pressure upon the midbrain and upper pons. If increased intracranial pressure involves a space-occupying lesion or results in asymmetrical edema, herniation—which will alter cranial nerve function—may occur. The alteration usually affects the third nerve, causing a fixed, dilated pupil. Alteration in auditory acuity would be an unlikely finding unless the increased intracranial pressure was the consequence of a lesion specifically involving the eighth cranial nerve or the auditory cortex.

492. The answer is A (1, 2, 3). *(Sabiston, ed 13. pp 1387–1389. Schwartz, ed 5. pp 1595–1599, 1720–1721.)* Although complete excision of a neuroblastoma is curative, in the presence of local invasion and metastasis excision alone is usually inadequate. Therefore, in most cases, treatment consists of surgical removal of as much tumor as possible coupled with chemotherapy and irradiation. Irradiation is usually directed locally to the tumor bed and to any sites of known metastases. Bone pain from metastases can be severe but may be relieved by irradiation of affected bony sites. Chemotherapy, usually employing a combination of agents such as cyclophosphamide and vincristine, has been found to increase survival in affected patients when coupled with irradiation.

Otolaryngology

DIRECTIONS: Each question below contains five suggested responses. Select the **one best** response to each question.

493. Which of the following statements concerning nasopharyngeal cancer is true?

(A) It has an unusually high incidence among Chinese
(B) It occurs primarily after the sixth decade of life
(C) It undergoes early metastasis to the lungs
(D) The treatment of choice is wide surgical excision of the primary tumor
(E) Initial evaluation should involve a biopsy of the primary and neck nodes

494. All the following statements regarding squamous cell carcinoma of the floor of the mouth are true EXCEPT

(A) it invades surrounding structures early
(B) it has a 5-year survival rate of less than 40 percent
(C) it metastasizes to bilateral cervical lymph nodes
(D) it frequently presents early as a mucosal lesion only
(E) it is treated with combined adjuvant radiotherapy and surgery

495. All the following statements regarding chemotherapy for squamous cell carcinoma of the head and neck are true EXCEPT

(A) preoperative (induction) chemotherapy can be expected to produce responses in over 75 percent of patients
(B) when a ''complete'' response to induction chemotherapy occurs, there is a high probability of local control and cure
(C) if there is no response to induction chemotherapy, surgical resection should probably be avoided
(D) patients with complete responses to chemotherapy do not require surgery or irradiation
(E) combined chemotherapy-radiation-surgery has not been shown to improve the cure rate for squamous cell cancers of the head and neck

496. All the following statements regarding carcinoma of the lip are true EXCEPT

(A) it is most frequently a squamous cell carcinoma
(B) it occurs most frequently in the lower lip
(C) it is radioresistant
(D) it is usually low grade and well differentiated
(E) it metastasizes via lymphatics

DIRECTIONS: Each question below contains four suggested responses of which **one or more** is correct. Select

A	if	**1, 2, and 3**	are correct
B	if	**1 and 3**	are correct
C	if	**2 and 4**	are correct
D	if	**4**	is correct
E	if	**1, 2, 3, and 4**	are correct

497. Correct statements about branchial cleft anomalies include which of the following?

(1) A fistula that lies between the external auditory canal and the submandibular region originates from the first branchial cleft
(2) The course of the first branchial cleft fistula is through the bifurcation of the carotid artery
(3) Injury to the hypoglossal nerve may occur during excision of a second branchial cleft fistula
(4) The internal opening of the second branchial cleft fistula is usually found in the maxillary sinus

498. True statements regarding cancer of the tongue include which of the following?

(1) Carcinomas at the base of the tongue are best treated by irradiation alone rather than surgery
(2) Stage I and stage II cancers of the mobile tongue may be treated equally well by irradiation or surgery
(3) Tongue cancers are relatively rare tumors of the oral cavity and are usually advanced to stage III by the time they are diagnosed
(4) Prophylactic irradiation of the neck nodes is indicated in patients whose primary cancer of the tongue is treated by irradiation

499. Pleomorphic adenomas (mixed tumors) of the salivary glands are characterized by which of the following?

(1) They occur most commonly on the lips, tongue, and palate
(2) They are rapid-growing
(3) They tend to recur if simply enucleated
(4) They present as rock-hard masses

500. Verrucous carcinoma of the buccal mucosa is identified with which of the following characteristics?

(1) It is slower growing than the epidermoid form
(2) It is associated with tobacco chewing
(3) It has a predilection for the gingivobuccal gutter
(4) It rarely extends to the mandible

Otolaryngology Answers

493. The answer is A. *(Schwartz, ed 5. pp 604–606.)* There is an unusually high incidence of carcinoma of the nasopharynx among Chinese. In the early stages of the disease, metastases remain confined to the neck. Diagnosis of nasopharyngeal cancer, which tends to arise in relatively young people, should be made by biopsy of the primary tumor. Biopsy of the neck nodes should be avoided because implantation of the tumor in skin and subcutaneous tissue may occur. Radiation therapy is the treatment of choice for the primary nasopharyngeal cancer. Cervical metastases that remain clinically evident should be removed by a radical neck dissection.

494. The answer is D. *(Schwartz, ed 5. p 596.)* The floor of the mouth is defined as that area of the oral cavity that is bounded by the tongue and the inner surface of the mandible. It is bisected by the frenulum of the tongue. The most common cancer of the floor of the mouth is squamous cell carcinoma. It frequently involves both halves of the floor and early in its course causes bilateral cervical metastases, as well as invasion of the surrounding structures. These tumors tend to be less differentiated than those of the tongue or gingiva. The early symptoms are minimal and are frequently ignored until there is pain and swelling of the tongue, which causes difficulty in eating and speaking. Thus, it is rare for a lesion to be found before it has extended beyond the mucosa. Radiation therapy is usually combined with surgical excision. The 5-year survival rate for patients with this tumor is less than 40 percent.

495. The answer is D. *(Erwin, Semin Oncol 12:71–82, 1985.)* Induction (preoperative) chemotherapy can be expected to result in response rates at or above 75 percent. Variously reported clinical trials have found complete responses in 25 to over 50 percent. Evidence also suggests that those patients with a complete response to either chemotherapy or combined synchronous chemoradiotherapy are likely to have long-term local control (‘‘cure’’). Conversely, those who respond poorly to induction chemotherapy have a bad prognosis whatever subsequent therapy is provided. Many workers now urge that surgical efforts be avoided in patients who do not respond to pretreatment since even heroic palliative surgery will not prevent early relapse. It seems clear that with currently used chemotherapeutic agents, there is an accelerated rate of relapse if the chemotherapy is not followed by surgical or irradiation extirpation of the primary site; chemotherapy should be considered adjunctive, not definitive, treatment.

496. The answer is C. *(Schwartz, ed 5. pp 588–590.)* The majority of cancers of the lip are squamous cell carcinomas. They represent 15 percent of all tumors of the oral cavity. Basal cell carcinomas of the lip occur less frequently. Over 90 percent of squamous cell carcinomas occur in the lower lip. There is a direct correlation between prolonged exposure to sunlight and carcinoma of the lip, especially in people with fair complexions. These tumors are usually low-grade, well-differentiated lesions. They spread via lymphatics. Lower lip lesions drain to the ipsilateral submental nodes, and upper lip lesions drain to lymph nodes anterior to the submaxillary gland. Carcinoma of the lip is radiosensitive, and treatment options include surgery and radiation therapy. Five-year survival rates for tumors less than 1 cm are 90 percent; however, patients with larger lesions with metastasis to lymph nodes have up to only a 50 percent five-year survival.

497. The answer is B (1, 3). *(Schwartz, ed 5. pp 1689–1690, 2118–2119.)* Branchial cleft cysts, sinuses, and fistulas are remnants of the first and second branchial pouches. The internal opening of the first is the external auditory canal; for the second, it is the posterolateral pharynx below the tonsillar fossa. The facial nerve may be injured during dissection of the first fistula. The second fistula passes between the carotid bifurcation and adjacent to the hypoglossal nerve. In childhood most branchial cleft anomalies present as a painless nodule along the lateral border of the sternocleidomastoid muscle. In adults, superinfection of the cyst or fistulous drainage via an orifice in the supraclavicular region may occur. Treatment is surgical excision.

498. The answer is C (2, 4). *(Ildstad, Am J Surg 146:456–461, 1983. Schwartz, ed 5. pp 595–596.)* Cancer of the tongue is the most common malignant tumor occurring in the oral cavity, accounting for slightly less than a third of the malignancies in the area. About two-thirds of them will present as early lesions in the mobile anterior portion of the tongue. Most workers in the field agree that for these stage I and stage II lesions, surgery and irradiation give equivalent results (45 percent 5-year survival) and the treatment, therefore, should be tailored to the patient. Failures are almost always due to supraclavicular recurrence and many recommend excision of the radiation scar and prophylactic irradiation of the neck nodes, particularly in the poorer prognosis stage II and stage IV tumors in the base of the tongue.

499. The answer is B (1, 3). *(Schwartz, ed 5. pp 593, 609–612.)* There are approximately 400 to 700 minor salivary glands in the oral cavity. Pleomorphic adenomas (mixed tumors) can occur in any of them. These round tumors have a rubbery consistency and are slow-growing; all are potentially malignant. Unless adequately excised, they tend to recur locally in a high percentage of cases. The sites most commonly affected by pleomorphic adenomas of the salivary glands are the lips, tongue, and palate.

500. The answer is A (1, 2, 3). *(Schwartz, ed 5. pp 597–598.)* Verrucous carcinoma is a less aggressive form of locally invasive buccal cancer than the usual epidermoid form. Its frequency is increased in people who chew tobacco. The tumor usually grows very slowly, occurs chiefly in the gingivobuccal gutter, and has a tendency to invade bone. It is identified by its characteristic exophytic white shaggy appearance. Wide excision is the best initial treatment for this neoplasm. Even though the tumor may regress in response to radiation, it tends to recur in a more malignant form with metastases. Cervical metastases usually are not present when the lesion is first diagnosed; it is only for the most highly malignant grades of verrucous carcinoma that radical neck dissection and block excision of the cheek are indicated.

Bibliography

Anderson JE: *Grant's Atlas of Anatomy,* 8th ed. Baltimore, Williams & Wilkins, 1983.

Anderson RJ, Potts DE, Gabow PA, et al: Unrecognized adult salicylate intoxication. *Ann Intern Med* 85:745–748, 1976.

Barnes RW, Marszalek PB: Asymptomatic carotid disease in the cardiovascular surgical patient: Is prophylactic endarterectomy necessary? *Stroke* 12:497–500, 1981.

Bergqvist D: *Postoperative Thromboembolism.* New York, Springer-Verlag, 1983.

Boucher CA, et al: Determination of cardiac risk by dipyridamole-thallium imaging before peripheral vascular surgery. *N Engl J Med* 312:389–394, 1985.

Braunwald E, Isselbacher KJ, Petersdorf RG, et al: *Harrison's Principles of Internal Medicine,* 11th ed. New York, McGraw-Hill, 1987.

Brooks J: *Surgery of the Pancreas.* Philadelphia, WB Saunders, 1983.

Catalona WJ: Current management of testicular tumors. *Surg Clin North Am* 62:1119–1127, 1982.

Colacchio T, LoGerfo P, Feind C: Surgical management of parathyroid disease: A review. *Head Neck Surg* 2:487–493, 1980.

Copeland EM III: *Surgical Oncology.* New York, Wiley, 1983.

Cox EF, et al: Blunt trauma to the liver. *Ann Surg* 207:126–134, 1988.

Cummings RA, et al: Pneumopericardium resulting in cardiac tamponade. *Ann Thorac Surg* 37:511–518, 1984.

Davis JH, et al (eds): *Clinical Surgery.* St. Louis, CV Mosby, 1987.

DeBakey ME, et al: Patterns of atherosclerosis and their surgical significance. *Ann Surg* 201:115–131, 1985.

Elwyn DH, Kinney JM, Askanazi J: Energy expenditure in surgical patients. *Surg Clin North Am* 61:550, 1981.

Emmett M, Narins RG: Clinical use of the anion gap. *Medicine* 56:38–54, 1978.

Erwin TJ, Clark JR, Weichselbaum RR: Multidisciplinary treatment of advanced squamous carcinoma of the head and neck. *Semin Oncol* 12:71–82, 1985.

Falcone MD, Nappi JF: Chemotherapy and wound healing. *Surg Clin North Am* 64:779–794, 1984.

Fidler IJ, Nicolson GL: The process of cancer invasion and metastasis. *Cancer Bull* 39:126–131, 1987.

Fischer JE: *Surgical Nutrition.* Boston, Little, Brown, 1983.

Fischer RP, Beverlin BC, Engrav LH, et al: Diagnostic peritoneal lavage: Fourteen years and 2586 patients later. *Am Surg* 136:701–704, 1978.

Freinkel RK, Cage GW, Caro WA, et al: Precursors to malignant melanoma. *JAMA* 251:1864–1866, 1984.

Gilman AG, et al (eds): *Goodman and Gilman's The Pharmacological Basis of Therapeutics,* 7th ed. New York, Macmillan, 1985.

Haimovici H: *Vascular Surgery,* 2nd ed. East Norwalk, CT, Appleton-Century-Crofts, 1984.

Hall EJ: Radiation biology. *Cancer* 55:2051–2057, 1985.

Hardy JT (ed): *Hardy's Textbook of Surgery,* 2nd ed. Philadelphia, JB Lippincott, 1988.

Howard RJ, Simmons RL: *Surgical Infectious Diseases,* 2nd ed. Norwalk, CT, Appleton & Lange, 1987.

Ildstad ST, Bigelow ME, Remensnyder JP: Squamous cell carcinoma of the tongue: A comparison of the anterior two thirds of the tongue with its base. *Am J Surg* 146:456–461, 1983.

Kohn HI, Fry RJM: Radiation carcinogenesis. *N Engl J Med* 310:504–511, 1984.

Landercasper J, et al: Follow-up on toxic shock syndrome. *MMWR* 29:441, 1980.

Landercasper J, et al: Toxic shock syndrome and multiple-system organ failure after breast biopsy. *Surgery* 102:96–98, 1987.

Lawrence PF, et al (eds.): *Essentials of General Surgery.* Baltimore, Williams & Wilkens, 1988.

Lindner DJ, et al: Long-term hemodynamic and clinical sequelae of lower extremity deep vein thrombosis. *J Vasc Surg* 4:436–442, 1986.

Lotze MT, Rosenberg SA: The immunologic treatment of cancer. *Cancer* 38:68–94, 1988.

Meyer HW: Pneumopyopericardium. *J Thorac Surg* 17:62–71, 1948.

Miller RD: *Anesthesia,* 2nd ed. New York, Churchill Livingstone, 1986.

Ngai SH, Mark LC, Papper EM: Pharmacologic and physiologic aspects of anesthesiology. *N Engl J Med* 282:541–548, 1970.

Pasternack PF, et al: The value of the radionuclide angiogram in the prediction of perioperative myocardial infarction in patients undergoing lower extremity revascularization procedures. *Circulation* 72:13–17, 1985.

Pontes, JE: Urologic injuries. *Surg Clin North Am* 57:77–96, 1977.

Recommendations for prevention of HIV transmission in health care settings. *NY State J Med* 88:25–31, 1988.

Rudolph R, Larson DL: Etiology and treatment of chemotherapeutic agent extravasation injuries: A review. *J Clin Oncol* 5:1116–1126, 1987.

Rutherford RB: *Vascular Surgery,* 2nd ed. Philadelphia, WB Saunders, 1984.

Sabiston DC Jr: *Davis-Christopher Textbook of Surgery,* 13th ed. Philadelphia, WB Saunders, 1986.

Sabiston DC Jr, Spencer FC: *Gibbon's Surgery of the Chest,* 4th ed. Philadelphia, WB Saunders, 1983.

Schwartz GF, et al: Clinicopathologic correlations and significance of clinically occult mammary lesions. *Cancer* 41:1147–1153, 1978.

Schwartz GF, et al: Significance and staging of nonpalpable carcinomas of the breast. *Surg Gynecol Obstet* 166:6–10, 1988.

Schwartz SI, et al (eds): *Principles of Surgery,* 5th ed. New York, McGraw-Hill, 1989.

Seldin D, Rector FC Jr: The generation and maintenance of metabolic alkalosis. *Kidney Int* 1:306–321, 1972.

Shires GT: *Principles of Trauma Care,* 3rd ed. New York, McGraw-Hill, 1985.

Shoemaker WC, Thompson WL, Holbrook PR: *Textbook of Critical Care,* Philadelphia, WB Saunders, 1984.

Starker PM, Gump FE: Gastrointestinal disorders. In Askanazi J (ed): *Fluid and Electrolyte Management in Critical Care.* Woburn, MA, Butterworth, 1986.

Telford GL, Quebbeman EJ, Condon RE: A protocol to reduce risk of contracting AIDS and other blood-borne diseases in the OR. *Surg Rounds* 10:30–37, 1987.

Thomas WG, Thompson MH, Williamson RC: The long-term outcome of Billroth I partial gastrectomy for benign gastric ulcer. *Ann Surg* 195:189–195, 1982.

Thoren T, Wattwil M: Effects on gastric emptying of thoracic epidural analgesia with morphine or bupivacaine. *Anesth Analg* 67:687–694, 1988.

Todd GJ, Zikria BA: Mallory-Weiss syndrome: A changing clinical picture. *Ann Surg* 186:146–148, 1977.

Torosian MH, Daly JM: Nutritional support in the cancer-bearing host. Effects on hosts and tumor. *Cancer* 58:1915–1929, 1986.

Townsend CM, Remmers AR Jr, Sarles HE, et al: Intestinal obstruction from medication bezoar in patients with renal failure. *N Engl J Med* 288:1058–1059, 1973.

Veronesi, et al: Thin stage I primary cutaneous malignant melanoma. *N Engl J Med* 318:1159–1162, 1988.

Walt AJ: *Early Care of the Injured Patient,* 3rd ed. Philadelphia, WB Saunders, 1982.

Walters HL, et al: Peritoneal lavage and the surgical resident. *Surg Gynecol Obstet* 165:496–502, 1988.

Way LW: *Current Surgical Diagnosis and Treatment,* 8th ed. Norwalk, CT, Appleton & Lange, 1988.

West JB: *Respiratory Physiology: The Essentials,* 3rd ed. Baltimore, Williams & Wilkins, 1985.

Williams GM: Food and cancer. *Nutrition International* 1:49–59, 1985.

Wilson RF, Murray C, Antonenko D: Nonpenetrating thoracic injuries. *Surg Clin North Am* 57:17–35, 1977.

Wiot JF: The radiologic manifestations of blunt chest trauma. *JAMA* 231:500–503, 1975.

Zikria BA, Budd DC, Floch F, et al: What is clinical smoke poisoning? *Ann Surg* 181:151–156, 1975.

Zuidema GD, Rutherford RB, Ballinger WF II: *The Management of Trauma,* 4th ed. Philadelphia, WB Saunders, 1985.